The Pilates Powerhouse

THE PILATES® POWERHOUSE

THE TOTAL BODY SCULPTING SYSTEM FOR LOSING WEIGHT AND RESHAPING YOUR BODY FROM HEAD TO TOE

Mari Winsor
with Mark Laska

DA CAPO PRESS
A MEMBER OF THE PERSEUS BOOKS GROUP

Cataloging-in-Publication data for this book is available from the Library of Congress
ISBN: 0-7382-0228-2

Published by Da Capo Press
A member of the Perseus Books Group
http://www.dacapopress.com

Da Capo Books are available at special discounts for bulk purchases in the U.S. by corporations, institutions, and other organizations. For more information, please contact the Special Markets Department at the Perseus Books Group, 11 Cambridge Center, Cambridge, MA 02142, or call (800) 255-1514 or 617-252-5298, or e-mail j.mcrary@perseusbooks.com.

Cover design by Alex Camlin
Text design by Jane Raese
Set in 11-point Janson by the Perseus Books Group

Winsor Pilates® logo and author photo on cover courtesy of Guthy-Renker Corporation
Geoffrey Rhue—Photo stylist
Elizabetta Rogiani—Clothing designer
Ted Davis—Photographer
Eric Bernard—Hair and make-up

19 20 21 22 23 24 25—06 05 04 03
First Printing, September 1999

Dedicated to
my mentor Romana Krysanowska
and to my mother, Ann Hanlon

CONTENTS

Special Thanks To

My sisters, Gwen Smookler and Phyllis Mazure. My niece, Mari, for all her support and love. Elliot, "Mad Dog" Jerry, Michael Stadvec, Ludo, Melissa, Jane, Carl, Arnold Rifkin, Danny Glover, Mel Berger, Marnie Cochran, and all the trainers at Winsor Fitness, especially Brian Fr., Dena, Jane, Kitty, Vincent, Saul, Dagne, Roger, Rachel, Cindy, and Veronica.

All of the faith, endurance, energy, intelligence, and "guts" needed to commit to this project, I owe to God.

The Pilates Powerhouse

I have been an avid exerciser for more than ten years, and in the past, I often found myself battling muscle strains and fatigue.

Mari Winsor has taught me that I can tone, strengthen, and lengthen *my body while at the same time treating it with kindness and respect.*

Thank you, Mari!

—COURTNEY THORNE-SMITH

Introduction

Joseph Pilates was a revolutionary force in the world of fitness. Amazingly, he began developing this scientific system of body conditioning over eighty years ago, and after decades of research, he compiled these findings to create the form of exercise that is so wildly popular today. As we approach the next millennium, Pilates® Method of Body Conditioning has established itself as both a concept whose time has come, and the most practical application of an exercise that blends East and West. Pilates represents the total mind/body experience that can be effortlessly fit into our hectic schedules.

Joseph Pilates, the inventor of this all-encompassing health and fitness regimen, was born in Germany in 1880. He was a frail child with serious health problems. As a young man, he became passionate about physical fitness as a way to transform his physical appearance and improve his health. As he grew older, he became an accomplished gymnast, boxer, and circus performer, and was also an ardent student of Eastern philosophies such as yoga and karate. He called upon all of his research, study, and expertise to create a complete regimen that combined East and West, gymnastic and yogic principles, mental and physical exercises that would strengthen the body and free the mind.

Word of Pilates's remarkable conditioning system spread throughout Germany. The Kaiser demanded Joseph Pilates to train his elite troops. As he was an ardent pacifist, he politely declined the request and left his native Germany for England to take a job in the circus. Just as he was reaching the peak of his career as a performer, World War I broke out and he was interned in England for the duration of the war.

As you may well imagine, a prison camp is most certainly the worst possible environment in which to maintain a healthy body, let alone a healthy spirit. Pilates, however, somehow grew stronger in these surroundings. He became very resourceful, utilizing any resource available to him. When people are first introduced to Pilates, they are confronted by an intimidating array of specially designed equipment. Joseph Pilates fashioned the predecessors of the apparatus from anything readily available—his bunk, the bed-springs, and a chair—but the real center of his work comes from what he referred to as "the mat work." It is precisely this mat work that is the sole focus of this book.

His fellow prisoners knew that he had discovered something miraculous. He began to teach this method of body conditioning to them, and to their delight, they began to thrive. Soon after, he began teaching his method to the prison guards. The guards found this method so successful that it became a mandatory activity for the entire camp.

For prisoners and guards alike, remaining healthy in these camps was an even greater concern than physical fitness. Disease was a major concern. As the most brutal war man had ever known up to that time was nearing an end, a devastating influenza pandemic spread across the globe. It is estimated that 20 million lives were lost in World War I, but this pandemic claimed over 50 million lives in just one year. In rural towns, it was not unusual for 70 percent of the population to die in this epidemic. In urban or confined areas, where the disease could be spread much more rapidly, these numbers were even greater. It is remarkable that *not one* internee in Pilates's camp died from the epidemic, and Pilates himself always attributed that amazing statistic to his method. This did not escape the attention of the British military establishment. Not long after, Pilates was employed to train the most elite cadres of British troops.

Joseph Pilates's notoriety grew during this period just after the war, and many performers and athletes turned to him for training. Among the many who sought his talent was the heavyweight boxing phenomenon, Max Schmelling. As Pilates was an accomplished boxer himself, he was able to lend not only his expertise and knowledge of the sport but also his revolutionary method of conditioning to Schmelling's camp. Schmelling became so enamored of Pilates that the two became inseparable friends. As Schmelling worked his way up the ranks, he was given a shot at a championship title fight scheduled in New York City. The financial opportunities for professional athletes living in America were much more plentiful, and Schmelling decided that it would be much more advantageous to emigrate. This move meant that it would be necessary to bring all of his promotional, business, and training staff with him. By this time, Pilates was a close confidant and a valuable member of his entourage but was reticent to follow. Desperate for his participation, Schmelling's manager agreed to finance a studio in New York, as a bonus of sorts for Pilates.

Pilates left his adopted England for a new land, a new start, and a new life. On his journey he met the woman who would soon be his wife. With her help and the backing of Schmelling's manager, Pilates set up his first legitimate studio on 8th Avenue in New York City. In almost no time, the studio attracted an eclectic and influential following. It seemed that the most famous and interesting people in the world made Pilates's studio their home away from home. Among the many devoted subscribers to his method were Ruth St. Denis and Ted Shawn, perhaps the most celebrated names in dance at the time. Through their introduction, Pilates soon took on students like Martha Graham and George Balanchine, the founders of modern dance. Graham and Balanchine became early pioneers of the Pilates method. Balanchine went so far as to incorporate, move for move, Pilates's mat routine into one of his most famous dance pieces "Seven Deadly Sins."

During this period, my mentor, Romana Kryzanowska, was introduced to Pilates by George Balanchine, and she began studying the Pilates method. She is now in her seventies, and because she has meant so much to me and this work, I have added some of her experiences so that you may see, first-hand, how this method has been passed from generation to generation. "When I was first introduced to Joseph Pilates," states Romana, "I had injured my ankle quite badly, and was not able to dance. Back then, there was no such thing as physical therapy or sports medicine, and the only alternative was surgery, and even that was primitive. Joe said, 'this is how it works, you sign up for five lessons, and if your ankle is not better, I will refund your money.'" Romana decided to give this man a chance. "My first lesson," Romana explains, "I thought this man was crazy. He had me doing exercises that were not specific to my ankle. How could this help me? After all, I was a professional dancer that could do all these marvelous things with my body. The last thing I felt I needed was more exercise." Throughout her first three lessons, she continued to ask what these exercises were for and why she had to do them. After her third lesson, she noticed that there was no swelling in her ankle, and that she no longer felt any pain. It was then that she understood the first principle of this work: "Circulation is what heals."

After this third lesson, she returned to ballet class. "I noticed something that was different, an extreme, in tune, sense of balance and strength that I did not have before working with Joe. I noticed an utter control, and I felt that I was master over every body part, and it would move wherever I wanted it to go. My leg was perfect and my work was better than it ever was. I have believed in Pilates ever since." She became so intrigued that she spent much time with Joseph Pilates. "He knew the inner workings of the body so well, and understood the dynamics of the inner world that we are just becoming aware of today. He was an almost magical man, perhaps the most remarkable healer I have ever witnessed that also had a very keen mind. He read constantly, and his studies of mathematics and the laws of physics are directly related to every single exercise in his method. You will notice that the line of the body is at a 45-degree (or a 90-degree) angle, that the body is perpendicular, convex, or concave. You will notice that you are either working with or working against gravity."

When asked what she would tell the person experiencing Pilates for the first time, Romana replied, "Externally, you will notice how dramatically your body will change, your thighs and buttocks will slenderize, and you will become more keenly aware of your powerhouse. This place that is like a wide belt around the middle of your body, will be relied upon more and more in every physical activity. Whether you are just sitting or walking, your body will feel lifted. As a result, you will feel uplifted and joyous. Even after the first time you do Pilates, you will feel buoyant. You will feel completely energized, grounded, and ready." Romana adds this story: "I have a female client who studied with Joseph Pilates and has been working with me since his death. She is now in her nineties. One day while she was in the studio, she lost her patience with me as I was trying to explain to a young man what Pilates was all about and what it would add to his life. She interrupted my explanation and put it to him in these words, 'It's like this, young man. I come here to get my fix. I'm going out dancing tonight. I need the energy.'"

Since the death of Joseph Pilates in the late 1960s, Romana has trained a great many people as Pilates instructors. "Quite early on in my training, Joseph Pilates said to his wife, 'You know, she's going to carry on my work.' This, of course, was not what I saw myself doing for the rest of my life. Joe proved that this controlled and fluid motion works marvelously to strengthen and to stretch the body. That is precisely what I wanted to continue for the rest of my life." The debt the world owes this woman cannot be overstated. She has single-handedly kept this method alive with all of its integrity intact.

The evolution of this form has altered slightly as a new generation of professionals have come to the work and have added an exercise here or there to develop different parts of the body. Joseph Pilates's work was preserved by Sean Gallagher, who founded Performing Art Physical Therapy/The Pilates Studio of New York. Along with experts such as Romana Kryzanowska, he is responsible for both the certification of teachers and the methods employed to instruct. As both a certified Pilates instructor and a practicing physical therapist, Gallagher has truly incorporated and integrated Pilates into modalities of treatment that health-care practitioners can provide and utilize.

I was first introduced to this work in the context of dance. The methodology was easily incorporated into the techniques and principles I had learned throughout my life as a professional. I had originally come to the work to offset the physical demands of my chosen field. At a time when I should have been considering retirement, I found that my body was getting much stronger, that nagging injuries and soreness no longer hampered me, and that my overall health was much improved. Lifelong asthma problems were significantly decreased by using Pilates techniques, and I found myself better equipped in my professional life. After only one class with the woman who would become my mentor, Romana Kryzanowska, I became her student and exponentially increased my respect for this work. As my understanding deepened, my professional career improved and, because of Pilates, I was able to dance professionally until I was well into my forties. The work became so inspiring that I began teaching it. Teaching the Pilates technique, especially the profound mental and spiritual benefits Pilates offers, became so rewarding that I dedicated my life to passing this knowledge to others.

It has been my honor to teach this method of body conditioning to literally thousands of people. In 1990, I opened Winsor Fitness in Los Angeles. The studio was an instant success, attracting dozens of high-profile clients. I have trained many celebrities and professional athletes. To them, and to their dedication to this work, I am deeply and profoundly indebted. The physical and mental changes have become so significant in their lives that they began speaking publicly about it. Over the past decade, some of my clients have endorsed their work with me in the media and this has significantly elevated the public's awareness of this work. This awareness has risen to such a degree that Pilates has become the "in" thing to do, reaching almost fad-like popularity. The intense demand for this work, along with the help of my great friend Danny Glover, enabled me to open a second studio on Los Angeles' West Side, Winsor West. Still, I could not meet the high demand for this knowledge. I was approached to write this book, so that others could benefit from this incredible method of body conditioning.

Pilates has completely changed my life. It enabled me to dance professionally into my forties, it has helped keep debilitating asthma at bay so that I am able to maintain a healthy lifestyle, it has helped me recover from devastating injuries, it has transformed my self-image and sense of worth, and it keeps me calm and centered every day. It is my greatest wish, that if I can pass on even a small morsel of the infinite benefits Pilates offers, that in a very significant and tangible way, I can help you to dramatically improve the quality of your life. It is my honor to be a link in the long line of teachers who have brought this information into our collective consciousness.

The Power of Pilates

"If you honor the spiritual and scientific basis of this technique, and give over all your concentration and incorporate the fluidity of movement, you will possess all the keys to bring 'Quality' to this method and experience the profound benefits Pilates offers."

—MARI WINSOR

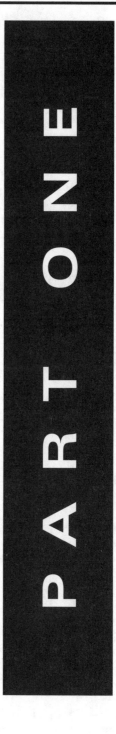

PART ONE

The Joy of Movement

*"I am really fortunate.
I get to spend my life helping people
transform their bodies and their lives.
They do it. I'm going to help you do it, too.
This work teaches you to accept and love yourself.
Only then can you really change and transform
your body. You need to find the joy of moving.
Then you can find the joy of you."*

—Mari Winsor

When most people make the decision to engage in regular exercise, they look at themselves with disgust and say, "I have to lose some weight," or "I need to tone these flabby muscles, so I guess I need to go to the gym." So they go to the gym, lift some weights, do some aerobics, and watch what they eat for dinner. After a while, exercise becomes mindless and boring, a means to an end. They don't even enjoy it. Exercise becomes just one of many tasks that have to be completed. If you are not enjoying it, what is the point?

The Pilates method of body conditioning is completely different. Instead of being mindless exercise, it is a very mindful activity. You must concentrate on what you are doing. This intense physical concentration forms what is known as a mind-body connection. With any movement or exercise, it is our brain that holds us back, not our bodies; our bodies are capable of seemingly impossible feats when we are faced with dire situations. It is our insecurities and thoughts of limitation that truly control our physical limits and performance levels.

If you are a sports fan, or you regularly play golf or tennis, you have heard about the "mental" aspect of the game. Very good players can make a mental adjustment in their game and become incredible players. Often it is this adjustment that separates professional athletes from superstars and champions. The same is true of performers. Competent performers can experience an epiphany, or breakthrough, that enables them to take their work to a different level. This is not a result of training or an improvement in their technique, but a mental adjustment, or a different understanding of what they do, that takes them to a higher performance level. In life, it is precisely this mental aspect of our "game" that leads us to fulfill our potential for greatness. The mindful physicality of this work frees and enhances our mental capabilities. This work can help us physically, no question, but the mental benefits that we receive that can be truly miraculous. I am certain that there will come a time in your own experience of this work when you will not be able to separate the two.

The mental aspect to this form of exercise requires practice, but will soon come to you effortlessly and consciously, and will have profound ramifications for you throughout your personal life. You will pass through several levels of this work, leading to you to greater and greater rewards. The first stage will be the most difficult. When you begin this exercise routine, you will note that you have an area of weakness that you need to work on. Recognizing this is critical. So you have a weak area. We all have them. The first step is accepting where you are at—right now. Do what you can, go as far as you can, and do the best you can right now—this moment. When you understand and accept these weak areas, you can go to work on improving them. Push yourself to improve and progress each and every time you perform this routine. With each victory, we encourage ourselves to go further. This progress becomes addicting, and brings with it a sense of empowerment. You discover that there is something that you can do to physically transform yourself, and that it is you who effects that positive change.

When we can physically conquer the limitations of our bodies, everything in our lives gets just a little bit easier. We become more comfortable inside our own skin. We enjoy being ourselves a little bit more. We accept our limitations at this moment, and look forward to improving. When we love another person, we love them for their strengths and their weaknesses. With self-acceptance, we can learn to love ourselves in the same way.

Literally every person who has come into my studio has commented on what a joyful and loving atmosphere they find there. This is no accident. Pilates allows people to be relaxed. Pilates gives people a sense of centeredness and a feeling of euphoria and happiness. This work is by definition life-changing—it will lead you to a quality of life that you may not even think possible.

At least ten times a day I find myself saying, "Pilates exercise can change your whole life." In this overly cynical age, I am increasingly amazed that this statement is true. This work can and will change your life. Pilates will help you to feel more confident, prepared to take on any challenge. It will help to reduce your stress level, improve your sex life. It will help you to be in the present, and enable you to have much more quality in your quality time.

The pride that you take in the physical is what I call "everyday pride." The efforts that you make to improve your physicality lead to a sense of self-assuredness, an ability to be comfortable with who you are, and inspire the confidence that by doing all that you are capable of doing, you are indeed a "success."

You never know what's going to hit you during the day. When you're clear and when you feel good about yourself, you're apt to make a better decision or perform on a much higher level. You're at work, for example, at your daily routine, when the president of the company comes in and asks you to do a special job; you've got to be ready. You may meet the man or woman of your dreams on the street. Some of the most important things we have to do and the most important decisions that we have to make come at us in the blink of an eye. There's no preparation time. Pilates will help you to be prepared.

I could tell hundreds of stories about clients who are more adept at meeting challenges in their lives because of Pilates. This work clears your mind, allows you to be truly present in your life every day, moment to moment. It helps you be centered and grounded, so that you are more effective, focused, and clear. You have a deeper understanding of your surroundings because you are calm inside and without distraction. You are ready for whatever challenges may come your way. During the 1960s, people did drugs to raise their consciousness. There is no drug that works as effectively as this workout to allow you to operate on a higher level of consciousness. I have many clients who liken this workout to a "high" of sorts. There is a mildly intoxicating, euphoric feeling. It is very addictive. You will find a way to squeeze Pilates into your busy schedule.

In this crazy world we live in, stress is a major factor in our everyday lives. Each time we turn on the news or pick up a newspaper, we are constantly reminded of the turmoil that we live in. But the relief from this everyday stress is oftentimes elusive. Some people may feel they need a drink to wind down from an exhausting day, but I personally feel that this workout is the perfect answer. It clears my mind and allows new information to come in. I do Pilates every day, so that I am better prepared to handle anything and everything that comes my way. Let's face it, most of us live in the proverbial storm. We all have to face life coming at us from every angle, and we just don't have enough time to get clear in our heads. Give yourself a great gift: that hour of Pilates in your day. You'll be more centered, and everything in your life will become easier. You are taking a break from the hustle and bustle. You can do an hour-long exercise and feel like a completely different person—without having to take a drink or a pill or any of those ineffective things we usually do to make ourselves feel better.

In this book we will discuss balance on many different levels: literal balance, as in not falling down, and the balance of muscular structure between a strong side and a weak side of the body. Balance also has a much deeper meaning in terms of your mental state and in your everyday life, however. How many times have you said to someone close to you, "I have to balance out my life"? We have to balance our time between work and our families. We have to balance our energy between those we love and the things we love to do. We need a balanced diet. We need to balance attention to our own interests with what may be good for those around us. When we achieve physical balance we do achieve a sense of beauty and symmetry, however balance in one's life is infinitely more beautiful. Innately, balance brings with it a natural harmony, both within ourselves and in the world around us.

Striking this balance gives our life quality. We find the room, and more important, the time to do everything that we enjoy. The benefits of performing this routine on a regular basis affect all areas of our being. We enjoy the benefits of self-confidence, a pride in ourselves, a readiness for challenge. The sense of clear-headedness and mental clarity it produces help us to be much more productive with our time. When we make time to work on our physicality, that time helps us to truly be in the moment. When we live in the moment, we are not ruled by our past, nor are we looking past the here and now for what is coming next. We take it all in stride. Being present helps us to be better listeners, to have a deeper understanding of our situation and surroundings. We become more perceptive and intuitive. We are more successful at work and at home. We are better spouses, better parents, better friends, and better people when we are really, truly present.

When most of us think about balance in our lives, our primary concern is almost always time. Most people never take time for themselves. They do and do and do for everyone else in the world, but when it comes time for them to do something for themselves, they are either too tired or there is simply no more time. If you know what I'm talking about, I want you to pay very close attention: I WANT *YOU* TO TAKE SOME TIME FOR *YOURSELF* EACH AND EVERY DAY! This time is not selfish time. It is in no way a negative thing. An hour of the Pilates exercises will be a very productive hour spent on improving yourself. If you think that this is negative in any way, I want you to turn it around a little. If you commit yourself to this form of exercise, not only will you feel great, but you will be much more capable of making those around you feel great. You will be much more effective at everything that you do.

The content of this book deals mainly with the transforming ability and power of the Pilates method of body conditioning, but the underlying message is that you have to move. Exercise. Do something. Millions of Americans take an hour out of their day as a break from their daily routine, or process through their daily grind, before getting on with the rest of their daily routine. Some go to the gym. Others zone out in front of the television, use yoga, Tai Chi, or meditation. This is the context in which you should put this hour of your day. You owe it to yourself to be the best that you can possibly be.

This is a treat for yourself, but it's not selfish. It is intelligent. It's intelligent time. It's an intelligent thing to do, because taking that time for Pilates on a daily basis makes everything else so much easier. As Pilates incorporates the benefits of aerobic and weight training, Tai Chi, yoga, and meditation, this hour will immeasurably enrich your life and will make you much more effective. It will give your life greater value. In the other twenty-three hours you will not only enjoy yourself more, but will find that you have more quality time.

We have discussed "quality" a great deal. As you can clearly see, the quality of your life can be dramatically enhanced through Pilates. For you, these qualities may be uncharted personal territory, or they may be exactly what you have been seeking. You very well may not be conscious of these changes in your persona as you become involved with Pilates, or you may have never realized that it is precisely these areas of our life that was your goal. The quality that you gain is derived directly from the quality of your movement. The notion of "quality" is truly being the best that you can be at that particular time. Quality of movement incorporates being in control, being aware of everything going on inside of your body, being keenly aware of where you are, and being present.

You will enhance the quality of your movement as you concentrate on how each movement flows into the next movement. The transitions are to be very smooth. I want you to think about this routine as if it were a perfectly choreographed dance piece. But please do not be overly critical of your work. Do not worry about doing something wrong. Just move through the routine. If you make little mistakes, you make little mistakes. Get over it. Improvement is on its way. Just keep doing the movement. You have to get stronger. You must never stop a movement because you feel that it is too difficult. If you feel that that's the case, simply modify the movement so you can continue. It's the continuation and the fluidity of the movement that's the most important thing. If you honor the spiritual and scientific basis of this technique, give over all your concentration, and incorporate the fluidity of movement, you will possess all the keys to bring "quality" to this method and experience the profound benefits Pilates offers.

When I first started this work, I did not get the mental benefits of this routine right away. My movements were mechanical, and I was just going through the motions. But my first class under the tutelage of my mentor, Romana, was a true epiphany for me. With Romana's guidance, I was able to glean the science behind the movement. As an example, let's say you have played football with the neighborhood kids since you were eight years old. At the level of eight-year-olds, the game is a very simple one. You get the ball, and all the other kids try to tackle you. When you get up to the high school level, you may be lucky enough to get a coach who is able to teach you the deeper meaning of the game. He shows you that indeed there is a science to the game. Every player is an important piece of the puzzle, and when each player fulfills his potential and does exactly what he is supposed to do, the outcome it is successful. The same is true of your body. Every part of your body is important. As the coach of your body, it is important for you to be connected and aware of every part, to be aware of every player on the field. When I first experienced this, I could feel it deeply and profoundly. I felt that all these moving parts had suddenly become one entity. I want you to experience that your body is one whole mechanism that is working for you.

Understanding the science of this routine will allow you to experience joy. When all the moving parts of your mechanism are working together as one, it is the most amazing and wondrous experience. When you are at peace with yourself and when your entire body is working in harmony, you will experience joy. That is the joy of movement. That is the joy of being you.

Principles of Understanding

The Science of the Art

"Pilates is the face lift of the new millennium."

—Dixie Carter

"Pilates has changed my life."

—Melanie Griffith

To not only experience what I refer to as the *joy of movement*, but to derive the full benefit that this method of body conditioning offers, it is important to be aware of certain scientific principles at work. Some people learn these principles in a logical linear fashion, some absorb their meaning on a more ethereal or conceptual level, while others learn by way of their bodies informing them—from the actual performance of the exercises. In whatever manner you derive understanding, it is important that you know the fundamentals of Pilates.

The actual principles are easy enough to comprehend. Basically, Pilates is a series of exercises or poses that are connected in a particular way to increase circulation and flexibility, and strengthen specific areas of the body. The routine, as a whole, brings the body into a state of harmony, so that all these areas are working together as one unit. Unlike most exercise, it is not how much, how strong, and how many, but rather an awareness of the whole body working in unison with proper technique that is the goal.

You are to be *present* for this exercise. Don't leave your brain in the locker room. Yes, you will be performing a very specific routine; however, it is the elements that you bring to that routine that makes this method valuable. As I stated in Chapter 1, with this form of exercise you are creating a certain level of quality in your life, and to achieve that quality requires your full participation. There are tools used in the physical work of this exercise that will help you derive the greatest benefits from the work, namely, breathing, relaxation, concentration, control, and a heightened sense of fluidity.

Breathing

Breathing is a bodily function that we perform whether we are conscious of it or not. In this form of exercise, the point is to be very mindful of the manner in which we are breathing. Each movement is tied to a specific manner of breathing. Correct breathing allows oxygen to nourish the muscles being utilized, and to release an array of nonbeneficial chemicals stored in the muscles. The chemicals released are related to pain and fatigue, and they are substances that our body is desperately trying to rid itself of. Not only is it necessary to take in an ample supply of oxygen, but we also must fully and purposefully exhale, or what I refer to as "wringing out the lungs."

Different disciplines require different methods of breathing. For instance, an opera singer breathes air in below the diaphragm, puffing the stomach out. A musician, especially a woodwind or brass player, breathes into the stomach and proceeds to fill the entire chest cavity and then the throat with air. For Pilates exercise, you may have to retrain yourself to breathe in a new way. When most of us inhale, we expand the top of our chest. We may think that this is a deep breath, but it is truly shallow breathing. An extreme example of this is when an asthmatic has an attack. Breathing becomes very labored, and air is gasped into only the uppermost portion of the lungs in an action that more resembles swallowing than breathing. What we need to learn to do is breathe into the back in the area that expands the small ribs. In other words, rather than having our breath expand the front of our chest outward or puff our stomach out, we need to concentrate on filling the bottom-most portion of our lungs. We should get the sensation that we are breathing into the small of the back. This form of deep breathing allows us to bend and move without restricting the amount of oxygen that we are taking in. The oxygen intake allows nourishment to travel to the muscles being worked. As we fully exhale, all of the unused gasses and nonbeneficial chemicals stored within the body have a route of escape. When these elements are expelled, we become more clear-headed, our stamina increases, we release the lactic acids within the musculature that make us feel sore, and most important, we become more relaxed.

Relaxation

One of the skills you will need to learn immediately is how to work out without creating undue tension in areas of the body that are not being worked. When people first begin this work, they simply work too hard. Some people, especially men, have been exercising in a manner that requires brute strength, and oftentimes it is the effort put forth that lends the best end result. In Pilates, however, just the opposite is true. You will be working a specific area of the body in each separate exercise (believe me, you will know where it is), and as those specific areas are being worked, it is your task to make certain that the areas *not* involved are working to support the movement. They are engaged, but not tense. For instance, when you are riding a horse, there is more to steering than merely sitting on top of the animal and leaving it up to the discretion of the horse to stay on the trail or not. You are holding the reins, your shoulders are relaxed but ready, your feet are flexed in the stirrups and waiting to signal, and you are squeezing with your legs. Your whole body is involved. With Pilates, it is the involvement of the entire body that helps to relieve tension in the body. After you finish the routine, you will notice that you have eliminated stress significantly on both the physical and mental levels.

Concentration

Often when we move, we are completely unconscious of the actual movement. The brain gets an image of what we want to do, and without us really paying attention, the body executes what the brain intended. For instance, there is a significant distinction between when you reach for your cup of coffee as you read the morning paper, and when you lift up a glass that has been filled to the brim. When a brain surgeon is working, you can be fairly certain that any movement that surgeon makes is deliberate and intentional. As our ability to concentrate on a specific area of the body improves, we dramatically enhance the quality of our movements. The movements you will be executing are very specific to an area of the body, and it is essential that you concentrate your attention to ensure that the specific area is working correctly. When we are mindful of our movements, the brain and the body work together harmoniously and effectively. Throughout the exercise portion of the book, I will not only provide you the specific areas of the body that you are concentrating on moving, but will give you some helpful imagery as well.

Control

Control is an essential key to the quality of your movement. With this form of exercise you do not have to overly exert yourself. You will not be flailing your limbs here and there; you will be moving with the grace of a dancer, having several parts of the body engaged in mindful movement simultaneously. There are never movements that are propelled by the momentum of throwing a part of the body. The exercise is executed by breathing, concentration, and stretching. When you first begin this method of body conditioning, you may go through an awkward stage. The exercises could involve parts of the body that you are not used to moving in unison. Have no fear, once you have the basic understanding of the move, you will be able to execute the movements gracefully.

Fluidity

The quality of being graceful while you perform this movement stems from the fluidity of one movement seamlessly blending into the next. I think of Pilates as being a perfectly choreographed dance piece, and to perform it with grace means to execute the movements with precision. Each movement or exercise has a specific point at which it begins and a place where it ends. However, it is up to you to blend these places into each other, and to make unrecognizable the points of reference within the whole. Even if you are instructed to hold at a certain point in each movement for a certain number of counts, that hold is not a place to stop, but rather a place where a stretch or movement continues, however unrecognizable it may be to an outside observer. Each exercise leads to the next. There is really no time when movement stops—the end of one movement is just the beginning of another.

Inside Out/Outside In

Conceptually, Pilates is an exercise that is paradoxical, or based on premises that may seem to be diametrically opposed. You will be working from the inside out, and simultaneously working from the outside in. You will be strengthening smaller muscle groups to support the movement and abilities of the larger muscles. You will be moving in a very controlled fashion to free your mind, and you will be using your mind to move the body. When you are finished with this routine, there will be a closer bond between these two aspects of your persona. You will feel whole . . . energized . . . powerful.

When the exercises are done correctly, you will be using your center, or *powerhouse*—your "inside"—to be the root of all movement. (This region of the body is so fundamental to the work that we will discuss it in detail in Chapter 3.) This center is the place that connects the abdominal muscles with the small of the back with the buttocks. From the strength of your powerhouse will emanate dramatic changes in the way you stand, move, walk, carry yourself, and physically relate to the world around you. You will be doing an external movement that will vastly improve your inner life. Working from the inside out, and outside in, will positively affect your mental clarity, the way you feel, your confidence level, your energy level, and it will also create a sense of tranquility and peace of mind.

Strength and Flexibility

This work is a combination of art and science. Like a perfectly choreographed dance piece, each movement fluidly melds into the next. Each exercise links breathing with strengthening and stretching. Each movement is designed to scientifically oxygenate, then stretch, then strengthen, and then restretch a particular muscle group. The premise of the work is to strengthen smaller muscle groups to support larger muscles. I'll give you an example. When you pick up a barbell to do a set of curls, the object is to isolate only that muscle and work it to exhaustion. Pilates actually develops smaller muscles that would go unnoticed with this isolation exercise. Imagine yourself doing that same curl with the same weight in your hand—only do it just a little more slowly and more controlled. You initiate the motion of your arm from your powerhouse, and you can now feel that same exercise affect the forearm, the shoulder, the scapula, the back, and the buttocks, while you use your stomach to support the movement. When the curl is performed in this manner, all those muscles are now working in conjunction and harmony with one another to perform the task. Your body is now working as a unit. The idea is to achieve your potential results more quickly, and without injury, by using all the tools available to you.

Freedom and Control

To hold up the spine properly, you have to strengthen your abdominal musculature. As we focus on pulling in the powerhouse, the place in our gut that links the abdominal muscles with the lower back with the buttocks, we can instantly feel a lengthening sensation in the lower back. If we pull the lateral muscles in the back down, the shoulders drop, the neck lengthens, and the spine becomes straighter. The more we concentrate on these body parts working in harmony with one another, the straighter our spine becomes. Remember the first time someone said, "Sit up straight"? We most probably jutted out our chest. This actually arches the middle of your back. The key is to pull inward into the spine by using your powerhouse. The result? Now your spine is supported. If you can learn to control this abdominal region of the body, and initiate movement from this place, a whole new world of physical movement and power will be revealed to you. This requires intense concentration, however.

If you can maintain your concentration, and be mindful of the manner in which you are moving, you can experience a peace of mind that is the ultimate freeing experience. To accomplish this, you should visualize your body being in wet, gooey cement. The cement does not bind you, and it does not inhibit your breathing, but you have to exert control in order to move. Your movements must not be quick or sporadic. You must, at all times, maintain control.

Pilates is a series of controlled movements done within the frame of your body, so that any movement will not pull you from the center of your body. You always want to be within the frame of your body. You maintain motion within the parameters marked by the width of the shoulders and hips. You never move your leg out further than where your shoulder ends. If you're lying on your side, you kick your leg forward and back, but you never take it higher than your hip. If you exceed these boundaries, you are inviting injury. Don't rely solely upon the large muscles to lift your leg up, because inevitably you will injure the smaller muscles that support that movement. Initiate all movement from your powerhouse. This will help to strengthen the smaller muscles and ligaments that support larger muscles and joints.

With Pilates, there is a routine or structure that will take you through each muscle group. The movements are slow and fluid, which demands that the movements be precise. This precision will demand physical control from your body. Like Tai Chi Chuan, these movements are not jerky but rather very fluid. The movements alternate between stretching and strengthening, while you breathe deeply into each pose. As in yoga, the combination of breathing, stretching, and exerting strength has a very soothing effect. Unlike yoga, the routine is much more active and nonrepetitive, and can be performed without a sense of boredom. The physical demands of the routine will enable you to feel a very deep sense of relaxation and a tangible sense of daily stress slipping away effortlessly. It is the precise control that you will demand of your body that will magically free your mind.

While you perform the physical tasks, you may experience a renewed creativity, and find that spontaneous images may pass through your mind. You may process through the nuances of your day, give birth to that really great idea, the pieces to the puzzle may all fall into place. . . . Who knows? This doesn't happen by way of a divine source of inspiration. It occurs by way of a mindful intention to move the body in very specific ways.

The Powerhouse

"Pilates gives me long, lean muscles and works deeper than any other workout I've ever done."

—MARISA TOMEI

The most fundamental and essential ingredient for performance of this routine is the ***powerhouse***.

The powerhouse is located in the center of the body. It is the exact point between the upper half of your body and the lower half of your body, between the right side and left side. Anatomically and scientifically, the powerhouse connects several large groups of muscles, and refers to musculature located deep within the abdominal region of the body. It is the place that connects the abdomen with the lower back with the buttocks. Joseph Pilates referred to this area as "the girdle of strength." Scientifically, these muscles are called the *rectus abdominis*, and refer to oblique muscles, and the *transversus abdominis*. When you see someone with highly developed abdominal musculature, or "the six-pack" as bodybuilders call it, you are looking at these muscles. The exact musculature we refer to as the powerhouse is located beneath these muscles, deeper within the abdomen, and is called the *transversus abdominis*. This muscle group, in association and conjunction with the *multifidus* muscle, is the anchor for the *erector spinae* group. The place where these three muscle groups—the *transversus abdominis*, the *multifidus*, and the *erector spinae*—connect is where you find the powerhouse.

In Pilates, all movements are generated by your powerhouse. This is where all of the energy that you exert comes from. Whenever you do an exercise, movement and control over that movement is always initiated by breathing into and pushing from the powerhouse. Always. This allows blood to flow more freely to the body and to the muscles that you need to work. Most of us who are unhappy with our appearance want to transform this exact area of the body. We want a flatter tummy and a tighter butt. Engaging in this work will absolutely and positively effect those changes by strengthening the powerhouse. Throughout the routine, there is almost constant initiation and use of the powerhouse; as a result, this area becomes much stronger and helps to reduce injuries. For instance, if there's an exercise that requires me to move from my hips, I have to push into my stomach with the abdominal muscles and initiate the movement from my powerhouse to move my hips. Otherwise, my hips take on the task of moving my entire body, and I can lock up and possibly injure myself.

Abdominal muscles criss-cross in layers across the front of our bodies like a corset, to act as a support for the spine. It is from within the abdominal region of the body, or powerhouse, that we support the spine and all of our major organs. Therefore, when we can strengthen this area, we also dramatically improve our alignment and posture; we can reduce or eliminate many of the problems associated with chronic pain; we can relieve and even reverse conditions that foster back and neck problems; and we may even enhance our overall health.

If your powerhouse is really strong, you can almost always eliminate lower back pain. A lot of people have lower back pain because their center is not strong, and they do not understand how to engage and utilize it. When they attempt to pick up a heavy object or participate in another strenuous activity, they will not utilize their powerhouse to initiate that task. As we strengthen the powerhouse, the bone structure of the body tends to be able to more fully support the weight of the body, which is better prepared to move, to exert itself, and to lift heavy objects. These improvements to posture will not only help relieve pain, but will increase your physical and emotional potential. You will learn that you can rely on this routine to mentally and physically condition yourself. From that center, you can control your own transformation.

> It is from the reliance and strengthening of the powerhouse from which you will derive *all* the physical, mental, and spiritual benefits of this form of exercise.

The powerhouse is not only key to your physical transformation, but it is also essential in developing a higher, more enlightened self. Physically, the area of the body that I have described as the powerhouse was essential to the evolution of our species. The entire development of man required strength precisely in this area of our anatomical muscular structure in order for him to stand erect and to walk upright. When he stood erect, man went through a process of mental transformation as well. Perhaps the missing link is really not missing at all. Perhaps it is within us. Perhaps when man began to walk, there was new information that he was able to process, or more tools with which he was able to process that information. Certainly when children begin to walk, it marks a distinct stage of learning. Is it possible that the powerhouse is another communication center for the body? Of course, we do have large brains, and this enables us to think and process information, but we receive information in other ways as well. We have the senses, we have instinct, we have intuition and perception, and we have feelings; these give us information on a nonintellectual level. This information comes to us by way of the powerhouse. The combination of physical and mental information processing just may be the reason why we, as human beings, have cognitive ability to reason, to emote, to express the profundities of our experience, to ponder the mysteries of our surroundings, and perhaps *why* we are the most intelligent form of life on our planet.

When the strength of the powerhouse can adequately support the spine, we begin to strike a balance physically. To achieve balance in all areas of our lives requires us to strike a center point. This chapter is specifically about the powerhouse, the exact area of the body that is the center. Much of this work is about finding your center . . . *your* powerhouse . . . a place of balance. It is a real and tangible place that you will become much more attached to as you participate and grow within this work. A potter has to center the clay on the wheel before he or she could successfully create a useful object. When it is off center, a washing machine will shake itself into a malfunction and turn itself off. When you are playing sports, you can be put off balance if you are not centered, and so it is with this work. Scientifically and physiologically, it stands to reason that anything operates better when it's operated from its center. So it is with your body and in your life. Pilates will allow you to develop that center.

The all-important task, then, is to find your center, or powerhouse. The notion of being centered is really to combine the physical and mental processes, to make a mind-body connection. Too often there is a distinction between mind and body. The brain is the center of all neurological activity, and the seat of our intellectual knowledge. The powerhouse is the communication center for the body. Being centered, or striking a balance between the mind and the body is a place that we want to occupy more and more frequently. Being centered helps us to be emotionally available, to be mentally clear, to be capable of accepting challenges, to become more intuitive and perceptive, and to be able to achieve our potential.

Emotionally, that center is the place where we operate best from. That center is the part that we love about ourselves, the person that we wish to be all the time. That center or powerhouse is the place where you speak from, where you feel emotional pain, joy, and elation. Emotionally, everything hits you there before your brain has a chance to process the information. Whether it is having a conversation that you don't want to have, or being asked to do something you really don't want to do, or having "a really good feeling" about a new aquaintance or business deal, it is the powerhouse that is always leading the dance. The information will eventually transfer up to the brain, and then you have to force the brain to get the powerhouse to relax so that information can be processed. But, with Pilates, more and more frequently, this will become a winning battle. The more centered I am, the more I pay attention to what's happening to my powerhouse, and the better my posture is, the more capable I am in every aspect of my daily life.

Mentally, the control that you exert over your powerhouse translates into a calm and clarity with which you can handle life's challenges and deal with them appropriately. We are constantly bombarded by negative stimuli. People project their personal baggage onto us, and they can be manipulative and pull us in different directions. When this happens too frequently, we lose focus. When we are centered mentally, we have the strength to stand up for ourselves because we are dealing from the truest and purest portion of our being.

As you get more in touch with this physical center, you will become more intuitive. When people say, "I have a gut feeling," they are really not off the mark. This center that you are strengthening allows new information to come in. It is the resting place of instinct. As you develop this area, you will come to trust this more. You will listen more frequently to that little voice trying to guide you. I have learned that this voice informs me daily, and all I need to do is trust that voice and be quiet enough in my center to hear it.

As you strengthen your powerhouse, you will, in fact, strengthen every aspect of your life. It allows for possibility to enter into your mind and your spirit and your life. People say that when they really get into Pilates, it changes their lives completely. Better things come to them. They have greater expectations. They are motivated to do things that they want to do. They are true to their ideals. They can express themselves more honestly and are more effective at communicating and in their professions. Personal relationships are fuller and more satisfying. The beauty of this form of exercise is that each segment is intended to strengthen this area. Each time you perform this routine, a new element will be revealed to you, and as a result, Pilates will never become boring or repetitive. If this routine becomes your exercise of choice, you will look upon Pilates not as a workout, but as a lifestyle that will continually transform the physical, mental, emotional, and spiritual aspects of your life. When you can find your center and learn to control it, this work, and everything else in your life, will become much easier to handle.

Doing It

PART TWO

Before You Begin

"Pilates is the only exercise program that has changed my body and made me feel great"

—Jamie Lee Curtis

"Pilates has proven to be the best workout for my body, mind, and soul."

—Elizabeth Berkley

No matter how uncoordinated you might think you are, or how insecure about your body you *think* you are ... All of that is about to change.

Doing Pilates, and doing it properly, is about going someplace that you've never gone before in exercise. Doing Pilates properly is about awareness. As you proceed, you will become keenly aware of the tempo and flow of the routine, and how one movement blends into the next. There are several areas of the body that you should be mindful of as you begin this routine, however. You will be developing your abdominal musculature and learning the correct placement of your rib cage. You will be developing smaller muscles that at this moment you may not even be aware of but that will better support the movement and usage of your large muscle groups. The importance of warming up your body will also be discussed. In doing this series of exercises, you will become aware that whatever your body needs most is what you will feel first. Most important, you will learn how to keep yourself motivated, so that you can benefit from all the life-changing attributes associated with this method of body conditioning.

When you are performing this routine, it is important that you frequently remind yourself of the importance of the powerhouse. All movement and control come from this place, and this routine is all about strengthening and utilizing this area. Remember, it's not just about doing crunches and getting your stomach flat. It's about using your powerhouse to support everything that you do. It is by strengthening the powerhouse that you get the abdominal muscles strong, contracted in, and cut.

As you strengthen the abdominal region, another piece of the puzzle begins to fit into place, and that is the proper placement of the rib cage. If you feel as if your ribs are protruding out, softly with your breath, let them fall toward your back. This lengthens your spine and you will feel more properly aligned. Another primary concern of proper rib placement is the area where the ribs meet the sternum.

We develop the abdominal musculature not only to look great, but also to act as a support system for the spinal column. As this support system strengthens, we go to work on lengthening the spine itself. Elongating the spine is vital in doing this work correctly, and holds the key to many of this routine's great benefits. The longer your spine is, the more efficiently your body operates. The more efficiently your body operates, the more efficiently your nervous system operates. The more efficiently your nervous system operates, the more efficiently your blood flows.

Energy passes through the vertebrae all along the spine. The longer your spine is, the more room you have between each vertebra. The more space between each vertebra, the more energy you will have. Try the following the next time you feel yourself getting tired—shoulders rounded, body slouching in your chair. What is happening is that the spine is collapsing. Now, take a seat on the floor with your legs crossed and start lengthening your spine. Close your eyes for two minutes. Feel yourself getting taller, as each vertebra lifts itself above the one below. The spine is a set of bones in your body that you can work on to improve your posture and to actually become taller. Lengthening your spine is essential to the transformation of the way you look and feel.

Soon you are going to be working some smaller muscles that you are not used to working. If you have ever taken up a new sport, you have probably said, "I feel like I used muscles that I didn't know were there." So it is with this. Even if you exercise regularly, the muscles I am talking about are not ones that most people pay close attention to. However, as you develop and strengthen them, you will become much more adept at any physical activity and far less likely to injure yourself.

A prime example of smaller musculature supporting large musculature, and where most people injure themselves, is the knee. The knee is one of the weakest joints in the body. A great many muscles support its proper placement, and several ligaments allow it to move in the way it was designed to move. When you say, "I threw my knee out," the pain that you feel may not even be in your knee. It is more likely that the pain is coming from the smaller muscles that keep your knee in place. Generally, the kneecap slides out of place because the ligaments aren't strong. With Pilates, you will be strengthening your quad muscles, your inner and outer thigh, so that those muscles will promote proper placement of your ligaments and joints.

Throughout your body, small muscles support larger muscles, and you will soon become aware that by strengthening the smaller muscles, you can lift more and move much more quickly. Your "game" will improve, and you will notice that when you do engage in physical activities, you will be operating at peak performance levels. You will have a sense that your entire body is working as one unit and in one piece of coordination.

Because my orientation to this work comes from the world of dance, I think of this as a ballet. This routine is a scientifically engineered piece of choreography, to work one specific part of your body after the next. Everything is connected. When you begin to understand how one move blends into the next, you can begin to concentrate on the tempo of the movement as a whole. In Pilates, there should be no jerky movements. Imagine yourself as moving through wet cement. The cement prevents you from moving quickly. Because you can't throw your limbs, you have to really concentrate on how the body gets from point A to point B. Then you realize that there are thousands of points that you must move through to get from point A to point B. Notice how moving through the cement creates a certain tension within the muscles: They aren't exactly flexed, but they aren't relaxed either. When you are doing this exercise, make certain that you engage the entire body in this way. Remember, your movement isn't necessarily "slow," but it is constant and controlled. And it should remain within the frame of the body. When you move outside this frame, you are far more likely to injure yourself.

If you do other forms of exercise, please warm up the body before you begin by doing the first several Pilates exercises. You will find that ten or fifteen minutes of various Pilates exercises will not only give you a good stretch and prepare the body for what it is about to do, but you will find that you are much more proficient at it. To participate in a game of tennis or a workout at the gym requires the body to be warm, with a certain amount of blood pumping through the muscles. Watch professional athletes. Before they even take the field for their introductions, they are sweating. They have warmed the body up. When you can warm up your muscles and ligaments, you can eliminate the risk of injuring yourself by about 90 percent. The beauty of this work is that it requires no warm-up period—the first few exercises of the routine are your warm-up, and it is perfectly designed to be a self-contained form of exercise.

As you begin, you will be keenly aware of the parts of your body that are weak and need to become more flexible. Whatever your body needs most, you will feel first. If you're inflexible, the first thing you feel is more flexible. If you need better motor skills, the first thing you will feel is that you are becoming more coordinated. You will also notice a vast improvement in your overall sense of well-being, and you will feel an almost spiritual connection to your body. You should feel rejuvenated after only your first workout. Your stress level will also be drastically reduced. When you experience stress, your muscles actually constrict, or tie up in knots around joints. This leads to backaches and to tightness in the shoulders, headaches, and many other illnesses. One of the aspects of this exercise program that you will concentrate on most as a beginner will be to lengthen these muscles away from the joint.

You will also test your will. If I told you that by spending an hour a day three or four times a week you could become physically fit, firm up those flabby areas, alleviate pain, become more confident, dramatically reduce your stress level, be more calm and approachable, become more intuitive, experience elation like you have never felt, and learn to truly and deeply love yourself, can you think of anything that would stop you from doing it? Would you like to transform your entire life? It will require some discipline, but you really *can* do it. You may not want to work out at first, but that will only last for the first few minutes. I promise to get you through those first few minutes, but I want you to make the commitment to bring yourself to this work. How badly do you really want to do this? The more you want to do it, the greater and more profound your experience will be.

Let's do it!

Pilates Mat Work for a Normal Healthy Body

"I have found Pilates to be one of the single greatest gifts I have ever received. It is the gift I give to myself every day. I pass it on to you, hoping that it will become a daily treasure for you also."

— MARI WINSOR

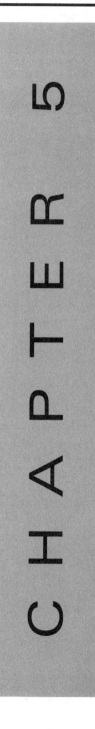

These exercises are for Beginning, Intermediate, and Advanced levels of proficiency. Please note that in the Table of Contents, and also in the top outside corner of each exercise, you will see one, two, or three dots, indicating the level of proficiency for each exercise. **Beginners** should perform all exercises marked with a single dot (•) in the order they appear. **Intermediate** levels should perform all exercises marked with a single dot (•) and all exercises that are marked with a double dot (••) in the order they appear. **Advanced** levels (•••) should perform *all* of the exercises in the order they appear.

If you are new to Pilates, start with the Beginners' routine only. With this routine, you will be working to strengthen the abdominal musculature and increase your flexibility. The Intermediate routine will work upon that acquired strength to coordinate movement and challenge you to develop even more strength. When you have graduated to the advanced stage, you will notice that each time you perform this exercise, you discover nuances that emphasize the profound ramifications of this method of body conditioning.

I have practiced this routine every day for well over ten years and have never found it to be boring or repetitive. Each time I do it, I feel better than before I started. I have found this method to be one of the single greatest gifts I have ever received. It is the gift I give to myself every day. It is one of the most precious and cherished of my possessions. I pass it on to you, hoping that it will become a daily treasure for you also.

All exercises should be performed on an exercise mat to ensure safety and quality.

This section is comprised of what Joseph Pilates referred to as The Mat Work.

Contents

The Hundred

With this exercise, we are increasing the circulation, warming up the body with coordinated breath and movement. When you are finished, you should feel warmth around the area of your heart.

Prep

Lie on your back.
Feel your whole spine meet the floor.
You should have the sensation that your spine is long and open.
Your arms are at your side and long against your body, and your palms are flat on the mat.

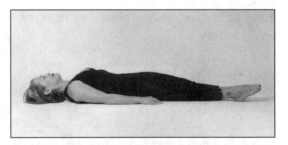

Ready

Bring your knees into your chest, and then stretch the legs up at a 90-degree angle.
Use your powerhouse to bring your chin into your chest; continue that motion as you continue to roll up.

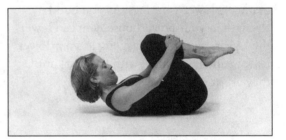

DO NOT lift the upper body higher than the base of the shoulder blades.
Continue to press your lower back into the mat and maintain this support for your spine.

Action

Pull your powerhouse into your lower back.
Inhale slowly through your nose for 5 counts
while pumping your arms
up and down on every count.
Your arms should be rigid.
Think of your arms as if they were hammers
vigorously pounding on a nail.
Exhale slowly through your nose for 5 counts,
continuing to pump your arms up and down.
Pull your powerhouse in.
Keep the arms straight.
Keep only your arms and shoulders involved
in the movement.

Repeat the cycle until
you have counted up to 100.
Relax completely.

NOTE: As you become more advanced you can
gradually lower your legs. As you build
strength in your powerhouse, you can lower
the legs in increments (as long as your lower
back maintains contact with the mat) until
they are at eye-level.

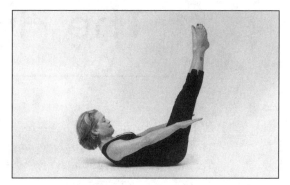

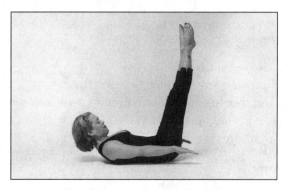

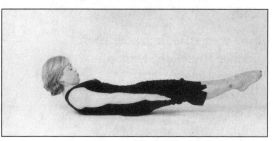

Roll-Ups

This exercise will really put you in touch with your powerhouse and will also give you a nice stretch in the hamstrings and spine. The powerhouse connects everything—from the fingertips down through your toes. As you do this exercise, try to feel that connection.

Prep

Lie flat on your back.
Feel that your spine is
supported and neutral against the floor.
Legs are together and flat against the mat.
Reach your arms above your head,
no wider than shoulder length apart,
with your palms facing upward.
Create a space between
your shoulders and your ears.
Relax your shoulders.
Initiate your powerhouse by sinking your
navel in toward your spine.
Feel long through your waist.

Action

While breathing in,
raise your arms toward the ceiling.
As you reach for the ceiling,
use the powerhouse to
bring your chin toward your chest.
Keep reaching through your fingertips.

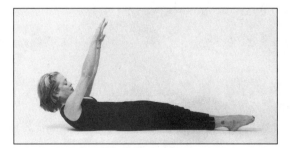

Make certain not to jut your ribs forward
to ensure the middle of your back is supported.
Breathing out,
continue reaching with your arms,
curling over,
as your fingers reach toward your toes.
Your spine does not straighten.
Create a "C" curve in your lower back by
pulling your navel toward the spine.
Continue the exhalation
until you touch your toes.

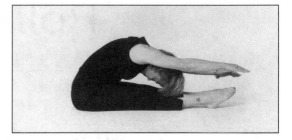

Breathing in, as you roll down.
Keep reaching with your arms,
keeping them at shoulder level.
Pull your powerhouse into your lower back
and draw your pelvis underneath you.
Maintain the "C" curve in you lower back.
Your lower four vertebrae
will make contact with the mat first.
Hold your breath at this point,
as you continue to curl down with control,
like a cobra, vertebra by vertebra.
Reach with your arms
to help control your roll down.
Now exhale
as you complete the roll down.

Repeat 6–8 times.

Single Leg Circles

In this exercise, you are loosening the hips and stretching the hamstrings. Despite the title of the exercise, I want you to try to trace a rounded triangle, an oval or football-shaped pattern using your leg. Keep the motion smooth. Use the powerhouse to support this motion, and lightly tweeze the buttocks for support, keeping both hips on the mat.

Ready

Lie flat on your back.
Your hands rest comfortably at your sides.
In this exercise, you are using your leg to trace an oval shape in the air.

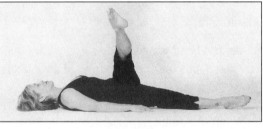

Action

Hug your right knee into your chest.
Keep the leg aligned with your hip.
Relax the right leg straight up.
Get as close as you comfortably can to forming a right angle with your body.
Cross the right leg to the left over your body, like a windshield wiper,
keeping your hips "quiet."
Once the leg is crossed, swing it down toward your left leg—like a sickle— by about 6 inches, and up toward the ceiling.
Stay within the frame of your body.
Keep the moving leg aligned within the frame of your shoulders, as you finish the "circle," and come back to center.
Repeat this motion 5 times. Now reverse the direction your leg is moving. Move the leg straight down, around, and up, and repeat the movement five times.

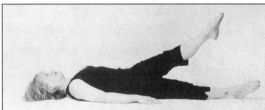

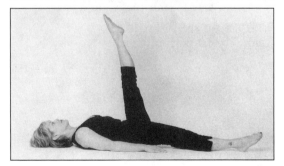

Exhale slowly.
Change legs.
Pull your left leg into your chest.
Extend your right leg out,
and repeat the exercise.

Rolling Like a Ball

This is like a little massage for your back. Your goal in this exercise is to not let your feet touch the floor. You will be coming to a point of balance right on top of your "sit-bones." Achieving this balance requires control from the powerhouse. Do not throw your body to come back up. Use your powerhouse.

Ready

Sit up and bend your knees,
as you scooch your buttocks toward your heels.
Hug your ankles,
and curve your spine gently over.
Bring your chin into your chest.
Maintain this position by
pulling your powerhouse into your spine, and
curving your back even more, so you come to
be in a ball-shaped position.
Make the letter "C" with your spine.
Arch your feet.
If you must, only your toes should be
touching the mat.
Maintain that position as you . . .

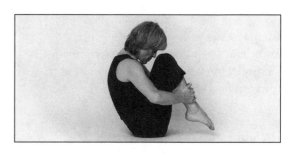

Action

Inhale slowly—feel the powerhouse.
Initiate rolling back by
bringing the navel into the spine.
Exhale slowly.
Use the momentum of your breath and
powerhouse to return forward.
Maintain the ball position.
Repeat 6 times.

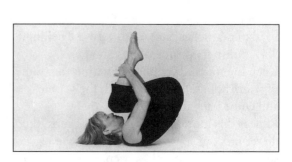

Roll-Over

When I do this exercise, I try to visualize my back peeling up and then peeling down. You should not throw your legs over your head. This exercise is a highly controlled movement. If you are moving slowly and controlling the movement, and feel pain, stop immediately. If you have a bad neck, you should not do this exercise. If your upper shoulders are very tight, sometimes this can be very helpful. The most important thing to keep in mind is this: You don't have to take your legs all the way over to the floor. Go only as far over as the stretch in your neck will allow.

Ready

Lie on your back.
Pull the powerhouse into the spine to lengthen your lower back.
Arms are straight down by your side, with palms against the mat.
Your legs are glued together.
Your neck is long.

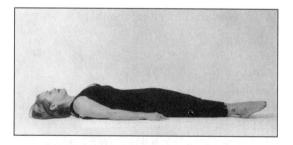

Action

Slowly bring your knees into your chest, stretching the lower back.
Stretch the legs straight up.
Use your powerhouse and tighten the buttocks for control.
Draw your legs over your head; keep your legs together as you go, and inhale.
Once your toes reach behind your head, open the legs shoulder-width apart.

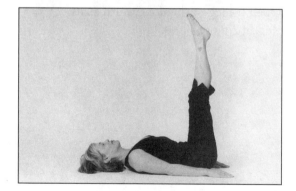

Exhale as you use the powerhouse to control
the rolling down of the spine,
lengthening away from the top of your head.
Keep your legs as close to your body as you
can until your buttocks touch the floor.
Keep your legs shoulder-width apart,
and lower them down until
they are at a 45-degree angle with the mat;
bring your legs together.
Repeat 2 more times.
Now reverse the movement of the legs.

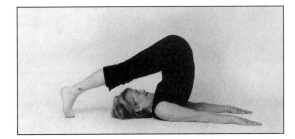

Instead of bringing the legs together,
open your legs at the 45-degree angle.
Use the powerhouse—squeeze the buttocks.
Keep your legs open.

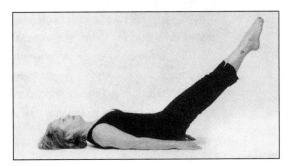

When your toes touch on the mat,
close your legs.
Keep your legs glued together, and maintain
control with your powerhouse.
Reach down with your fingers,
pull your shoulders down.
Roll down, vertebra by vertebra,
until your legs are at a 45-degree angle.
Open the legs a shoulder-width apart.
Repeat 2 more times.

Single Leg Stretch

This exercise is designed to work on your coordination, relax the hip flexors, and link breath to movement. As you concentrate on the powerhouse initiating this movement, you will begin to feel a strengthening in your abdominal muscles. Keep your shoulders square. The only parts of your body that should move are your arms and legs.

Prep

Lie flat on your back.
Your legs are extended directly out of your hips and are relaxed flat against the mat.
Your arms rest down against your body, with your palms flat on the mat.

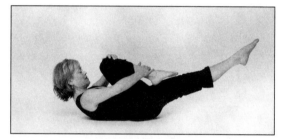

Action

Inhale slowly.
Lift your chin toward your chest.
Use your powerhouse to raise your head and shoulders off the mat.
Simultaneously bring your right knee into your chest and put your right hand on your right ankle, while your left hand is placed atop the inside of your right knee.
Relax your shoulders and open your elbows.
Relax your ankle.
Tug on the bent leg twice,
breathing out as you go.

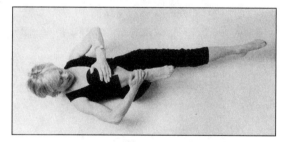

Now, switch legs.
Left hand to left ankle,
Right hand atop the inside of your left knee.
Keep your leg in alignment with the hip.
Tug twice, and switch.

Contract the powerhouse in as you exhale;
engage your stomach muscles at all times.
Repeat 8–12 times.

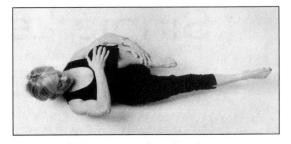

Double Leg Stretch

You will be folding and unfolding the body. The powerhouse contracts in and you fold. Imagine a comet hitting the earth, sucking everything into the hole its impact leaves on the surface. That's what your body is doing. The comet hits your powerhouse—you fold in.

Ready

Glue your legs together.
Bring your knees in toward your chest.
Hug your ankles gently.
Use the powerhouse to
lift your chin to your chest.
Exhale slowly for three counts,
contract your powerhouse further
by pressing the belly button toward the spine.

Action

As you inhale,
lengthen your legs
and lift them up toward the ceiling.
Bring your arms up, straight and long,
until they are even with your ears.
Your shoulders lift off the mat.
Your lower back remains flat on the floor.
Your chin reaches toward your chest.

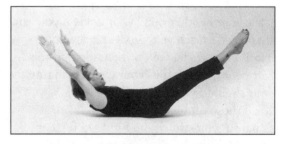

As you exhale,
sweep your arms around by your sides.
Using your powerhouse, slowly draw your legs
toward your abdomen, and hug your knees.
Hold.

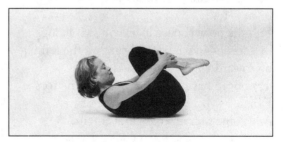

Using the powerhouse, stretch
your limbs away from your torso
and pull the limbs back in.
Reach. Fold. Hug.

Repeat 6–10 times.

Single Straight Leg

This exercise is designed to increase flexibility in your legs, especially in your hamstrings, and to strengthen your abdominal muscles. The straighter the legs, the more you will feel this in your abdominal muscles (abs).

Ready

From the Double Leg Stretch,
bring your right leg straight up,
until it is perpendicular to the mat.
Extend your left leg straight out,
like an arrow coming out of the hip socket,
until it is 2 or 3 inches off the mat.

Action

Inhale as you reach your arms up;
place your hands around your ankle if you can.
If you can't reach your ankle, place your
hands around your calf or behind your knee.
Lift your head-chin to your chest, bringing
your shoulders off the mat.
Keep those shoulders down.
Exhale as you stretch the right leg further
by tugging the leg toward you twice and
pulse—1, 2.
Pull the powerhouse in as you switch legs
in a scissor-like motion, bringing the left leg
up toward your body.
Try not to have any movement in the torso.
Exhale as you pulse your left leg twice.
Add some tempo to the movement.
Make it vigorous. Keep your torso still.

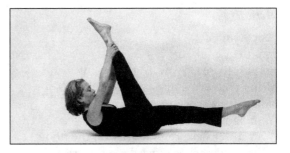

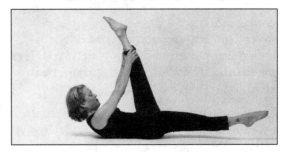

Inhale every 2 sets, and exhale every 2 sets.
Repeat at least 10 times.

Double Straight Leg

This exercise is designed to create strength and power within the powerhouse. Lower your legs only as far as you can without your lower back losing contact with the mat.

Ready

After you have completed the
Single Straight Leg,
bring your hands behind your head.
DO NOT CLASP YOUR HANDS—
either put one hand under the other or
let the fingertips touch.
Now rest your head into your hands.
Use your powerhouse to
bring your chin toward your chest so that
your shoulders are off the mat.
Both legs are straight up,
perpendicular to the mat.
Your lower back is pressed against the mat.

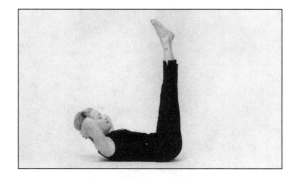

Action

Inhale as you glue your legs together, and
then reach your legs down slowly.
The legs go down as far as they can
without the lower back coming off the mat.
Take two counts to bring them down,
and one count to bring them up.
Your abdominal muscles guide the legs by
contracting down toward the spine as you
bring your legs back up.
Repeat 10 times.

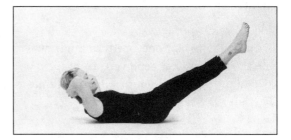

The Criss-Cross

The Criss-Cross is great for your abdominals. You should really begin to feel your abdominals working, especially if you begin by going very slowly. As one side of your body contracts, the other is reaching back into a stretch. This oppositional movement works the abdominal muscles diagonally.

Prep

From the Double Straight Leg,
bring both knees into the chest.
Extend your left leg up toward the ceiling,
making certain that your lower back
is pressed into the mat.
Your ankles are relaxed but not loose.
Your head and shoulders remain off the mat.
One hand is over the other behind your head.
Your elbows are open and should be extended
straight out from your ears.

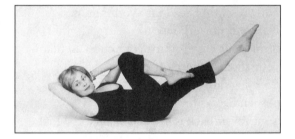

Action

Begin by moving slowly.
Breathing in, count one-one thousand, two-
one thousand as you bend your right leg
toward the middle of your right collarbone.
The left leg extends from your hip
at a 45-degree angle.
From the waist, use the powerhouse to twist
the torso to the right.
Your torso should move as one unit.
Look at your right elbow as it stretches past
your ear. The inside of your left elbow
reaches toward your right knee.

Hold for 2 counts.

Reverse.

Repeat 3 more times.

Double the tempo on the next 4 repetitions.
The small of your back should be pressed
against the floor.
Glue your butt to the floor
and don't rock your hips.
Double the tempo on the next 4 repetitions.
(Move to the tempo of "God Bless America.")

Spine Stretch Forward

This exercise provides a nice stretch for the entire back. You can really create some space between the vertebrae—this creates a tactile sensation of lengthening the spine. The key to performing this exercise correctly is to contract the powerhouse into the spine and intensify that contraction throughout the exercise.

Ready

Sit up.
Open the legs shoulder-width apart.
Extend the arms forward like you are sleepwalking.
Use the powerhouse to lengthen your spine, and lift your chest.

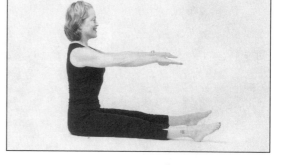

Action

While inhaling,
contract the powerhouse into your spine.
Starting with your head, roll down.
Continue the contraction until you are making a "C" with the spine.
Maintain this "C" curve and feel like you are rounding over a beach ball.
Exhale.
Your arms are in the sleepwalking position.
Reach the upper portion of your torso forward while maintaining your contraction.

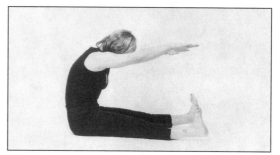

Your hip bones
should be over your "sit-bones."
Your buttocks are glued to the floor.

Inhale.
Roll back up.
Sit up tall.
Exhale.
Repeat 3 times.*

*After completing this exercise, you may want
to stretch your back by reaching your hands
forward over your feet.

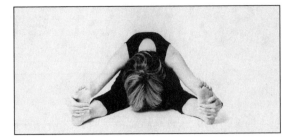

Corkscrew

There are three levels for this exercise. Only do the first portion of the exercise as you begin; as you become more proficient add the second and then the third as you reach advanced levels.

Ready

From the Spine Stretch Forward,
roll down to the mat vertebra by vertebra
until you are lying flat on your back.
Your arms are straight down by your sides,
with your palms flat against the mat.
Lift your legs toward the ceiling, keeping the
small of your back pressed against the mat.

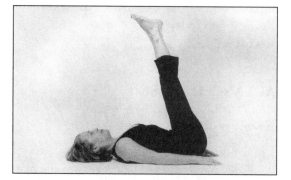

Action

Glue your legs together.
Initiating from the powerhouse,
move the legs to your right in a clockwise
motion;
outline a circle the size of a large pizza with
your toes.
Inhale at 12:00—exhale at 6:00.
Now reverse the circle.

Repeat 3 times.

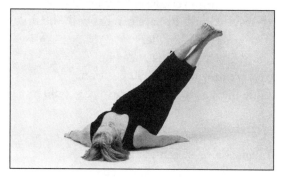

INTERMEDIATE LEVEL

At this level the circle gets a bit wider.

Action

Inhale as you
circle your legs around to the left.
When you reach the 9:00 position,
your right hip lifts off the mat.
Exhale as you continue the circle.
The hips meet the mat at 6:00.
When you reach the 3:00 position, your left
hip lifts off the mat. Come back to center.
Reverse the circle.
Repeat 3 times.

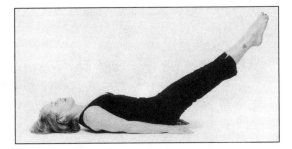

ADVANCED LEVEL

Ready

Lie flat on your back.
Arms against your sides, palms against the mat.
Using your powerhouse, lift your legs over
your head until they are parallel with the floor.
The arms and shoulders
act like a tripod to balance you.
You are now in the 12:00 position.
Glue the legs together. Relax the shoulders.

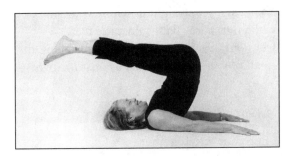

Action

Inhale as you sweep your legs
to the right as far as they'll go,
rolling onto the right hip (3:00).
At 6:00, the feet are 5 inches above the mat.
Exhale as you roll onto the left hip, sweeping
the legs as far as they will go to the left,
controlling the circular motion until you
come back to center (12:00).
Inhale and reverse the circle.

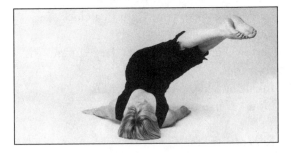

Repeat each stage 3 times.

The Saw

This exercise will stretch your hamstrings and your entire side from the waist up. Keep your buttocks equally and firmly planted on the mat to maximize this stretch.

Prep

Lift up from the powerhouse and sit up tall.
Your legs should be long against the mat,
shoulder-width apart, with your
kneecaps facing the ceiling.
Extend your arms directly to the side
like wings,
keeping them in your peripheral sight.
Pull the powerhouse into your lower back
and lift your chest.

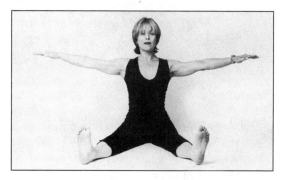

Action

Exhale as you glue your buttocks to the floor,
and use your powerhouse to
twist slowly to the right.
Twist from your waist, not from the hips.
Reach your left pinky
toward your right little toe.
Stretch your torso toward the right leg.
Your head should reach over your right knee.
Relax your neck,
and keep your opposite hip down.
Exhale slowly
and perform three saw-like pulses.
Saw that little toe off.
Stretch from your waist.
Complete the exhalation.
From the powerhouse,
inhale, roll up and return to center.
Repeat on your left side.

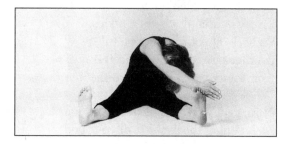

Repeat 4 sets.

Open Leg Rocker

This exercise is especially great for abdominal control. It will feel like a massage on the spine. This position demands that you keep your arms and legs straight.•You should not have the sense that you're rolling back on your head, but should let the head gently touch the floor. When you reach the intermediate stage, only do the "Ready" position; as you become more advanced, include the "Action" portion.

Ready

From The Saw, bend your right knee.
Slide your right hand down to your ankle.
Do the same on your left side.
The bottoms of your feet
should touch each other.
Place your hands on your ankles.
Sit back on your buttocks until
your feet are off the ground and
your toes are pointed toward the mat.

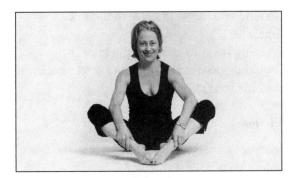

Now, gently test the flexibility of your legs.
Maintaining the position of your body,
pull your powerhouse in tightly as you
stretch your right leg out
until it is as straight as you can get it.
Now repeat with the left leg.
If this feels good,
repeat 2 times for each leg.

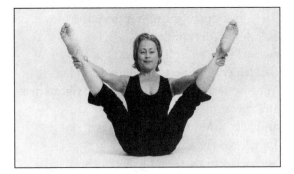

Straighten both legs out.
Pull in your powerhouse even further.
You are now balanced on your "sit-bones" in
the position of an archer's bow.

Action

From this position,
drop your chin toward your chest
and gently roll back,
pressing the powerhouse in.
Don't go back with such force
that you roll onto your head.
The powerhouse pushes you back up.
Only go down as far as you can come back up.
Keep your arms and legs straight.

Repeat 6 times.

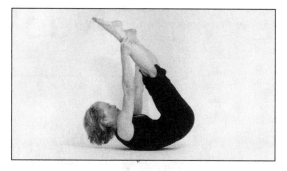

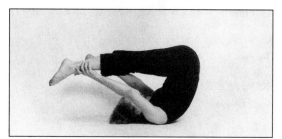

Neck Roll

You have been working your abdominal muscles really hard, so now it is time to perform an exercise that gives them a little stretch to say "Thank You." This will also give your neck a chance to stretch and relax, warming it up and loosening it for what is to come.

Prep

Release the body down to the mat.
Gently roll over onto your stomach.

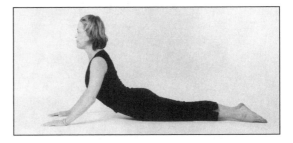

Action

Bring your hands
directly beneath your shoulders.
Glue your upper thighs to the mat.
Push up.
Arch your back as much as you can.
Pull your shoulders down.
Stay there.

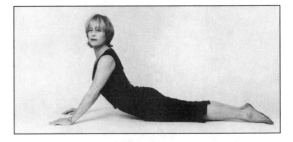

Look slowly to your right.
Come back to center.
Look slowly to your left.
Repeat.

Tilt your head toward your right shoulder
and circle your head around, with the crown
of your head leading the way.
Reverse the circle.
Repeat 2 times.

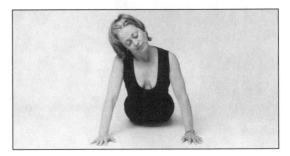

Single Leg Kick

I call this exercise the sphinx because of the position you are in.
This movement is very precise, so use the powerhouse to move your legs.
When your legs come up, be careful not to throw them toward the buttocks—
they move swiftly but with control. When your legs come down, utilize the
powerhouse to provide resistance.

Ready

Lie on your stomach and bend your arms.
Your elbows should be
directly beneath your shoulders,
with your hands closed in a fist.
Lift your sternum and chest.
Look straight ahead.
Your legs should be flat against the mat.

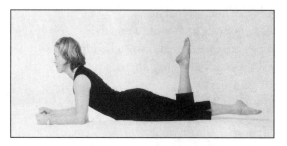

Action

Bending your right leg,
reach your heel toward your buttocks.
Pulse twice.
Relax your right leg to neutral, as you
bend your left leg, and
reach the heel toward the buttocks,
to pulse twice.
Pull your powerhouse into your spine.
Tighten up your buttocks.
Don't move your hips.

Do 5 sets.

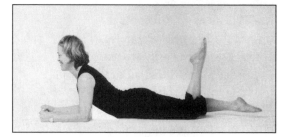

Double Leg Kick

This exercise lends a nice stretch for the abdominal muscles and lower back. You may open your legs a bit for this exercise, but no further than the width of your hips. If you have a bad back, this may not be the exercise for you.

Ready

Lie on your stomach
with your head facing to one side.
Legs are together and stretched long.
Clasp your hands together behind the small
of your back.

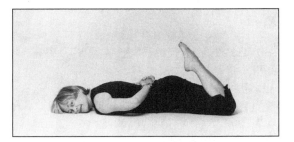

Action

Glue your legs together.
Knees bend as your feet reach
toward the buttocks and pulse twice.
Your legs stretch backward as you lift
your arms above the small of your back,
reaching toward your feet.
Keep your neck as long as can as you
raise your sternum up even further.
The crown of your head
continues to lift toward the ceiling.
Relax down to the mat.
The opposite cheek now rests
on the mat.
Repeat 3 times.

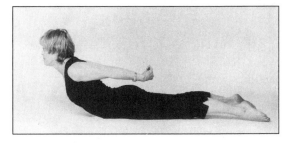

Swimming

This exercise really works on your coordination because you will be moving several parts of your body simultaneously. Work slowly and meticulously as you begin this exercise, and then pick up the tempo.

Ready

Lie on your stomach.
Arms are stretched in front of you.
Legs are together and extended from the hip.

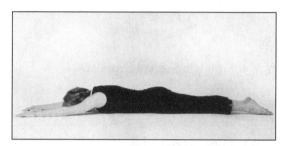

Action

Lift your head upward, and
lift your right arm and your left leg
as high in the air as you can.
Now switch.
Lift your left leg and your right arm up.
Lift them as far as you can and switch.
Now do it double time.
Alternate the arms and legs.
The movement is controlled and even.

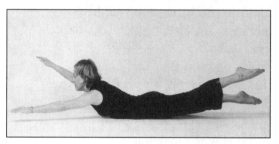

Inhale on 5 movements.
Exhale on 5 movements.
Don't stop or hold.
Don't let your feet or arms touch the mat.
Do 1 set of 20.

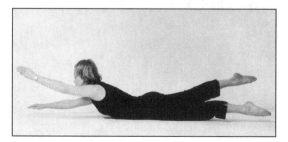

Little Piece of Heaven

My mentor, Romana, named this exercise. We have really been arching and working the lower back, and now it is time to give that area a little reward. If your knees hurt when you are rounded over, simply place a pillow between your buttocks and your heels.

Ready

You are still lying on your stomach.

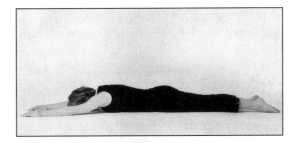

Action

Use your hands and arms to push yourself back onto your heels until you are kneeling with your back rounded over.
Focus on the mat.
Extend your arms long in front of you.
Push your hips to your heels for a deep lower back stretch.
Breathe slowly and deeply.
Rest the back.

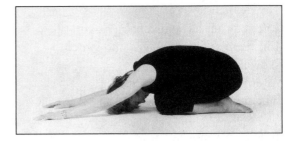

Neck Pull

This exercise is fantastic for building strength in the powerhouse. If you can remember to pull your lateral muscles in the back down, it will not only make the exercise easier to execute, but will prevent undue shoulder tension, provide you with additional length in your spine, and insure proper alignment.

Ready

Lie flat on your back, ribs relaxed,
belly button pressing down into your spine.
Touch your fingerstips behind your head.
Your elbows are relaxed against the floor.
Pull your shoulders down.
Pull your powerhouse in.
Lengthen through your spine.

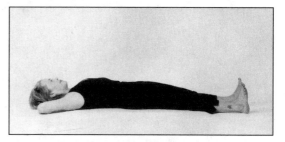

Action

Flex your feet.
Keep your legs hip-width apart.
Inhale as you lift up your head, and
bring your chin to your chest.
Continue rolling up, pulling the rib cage in,
and keep reaching with the legs.
Roll over all the way until
the elbows are pointed down to the floor.
As you sit, open your elbows to the side,
feel lifted,
and make your waist as tiny as you can.

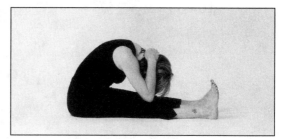

You are now sitting up tall.
Keep your back straight,
and lean back 2 inches.
Now contract in the belly button toward the
spine to roll the rest of the way down,
lengthening and reaching the legs as you go.

Repeat 5 times.

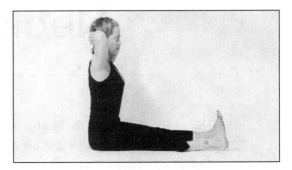

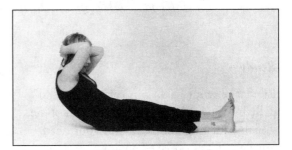

Spine Twist

The purpose of this exercise is to loosen the spine and increase flexibility in the hips and waist. To get the most out of this exercise, initiate the movement of twisting only from your waist. You will be watching the hand that is moving back. The motion is like sweeping back a circular shower curtain. Don't make the mistake of letting that moving hand initiate the twist.

Ready

You are sitting tall with your legs
extended straight out from your hips.
Your arms are extended
straight out to the side.
Feel that your chest is lifted.
Pull the shoulders down.
Your neck is long.

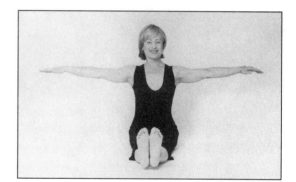

Action

The only parts of your body that are moving
are your waist and your neck.
Inhaling,
slowly twist from the waist to your right.
Your focus should be fixed
on your right hand.
The left hand comes forward.
Ideally, when you have completed the twist,
both of your hands should be
in a straight line.

Twist as far as you comfortably can.
Exhaling, twist from the waist
and slowly come back to center.
Inhale as you twist to the left.
Switch and repeat.

Do 3 sets.

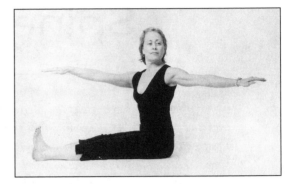

The Jackknife

The Jackknife provides an amazing stretch for the vertebrae, and it is also fantastic for strengthening your powerhouse. If there is too much pressure and tension on your arms and shoulders while doing the exercise, then you're defeating its purpose. In other words, don't let your arms do all the work; use them for balance, and let the powerhouse do the rest. I do not recommend this exercise if you have a bad neck or a bad lower back.

Ready

Lie on your back.
Your legs are extended straight out
from your hips.
The powerhouse is pulled in, and
your lower back is long against the mat.
As you reach the legs down from the hips
toward the toes, you want to feel energy all
the way from the hips to the toes.

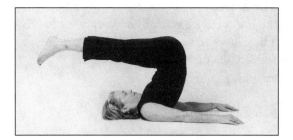

Action

Pull the powerhouse in toward your spine and
put a little bit of pressure on your arms.
Use the powerhouse
to bring your legs up over your head
(don't go any lower than parallel to the floor).

Now push your hips forward as your legs
lengthen up to the ceiling.
Your toes should now be reaching
toward the ceiling.
You are now in a shoulder stand.
The weight of your body rests on your
shoulders and not your neck.
Push your hips forward as much as you can,
so that there is a straight line
between your hips and your feet.

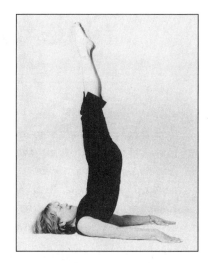

From that position, lower your feet slightly
toward your head, and use the powerhouse to
roll down vertebra by vertebra to feel a nice
stretch through your spine.
The harder you pull in the powerhouse,
the less pressure you will have on your hands.
The slower you can move, the more you will
feel a really nice stretch between the
vertebrae.

Repeat 3 times.

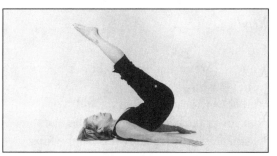

Side Kick Series

The only portions of your body that should move throughout this exercise series are from your hip down. You should utilize the powerhouse to hold your torso still and fixed. In this series, during which you will be lying on your side, body positioning is a key element in executing these exercises correctly. Your upper hip must remain directly on top of the other hip. It should not become displaced because of the movement. The torso should remain straight, long, and strong. This is a great exercise for the buttocks, hips, and thighs. Begin on your right side. **Go through this entire series on your right side, then roll over and go through it on your left side.**

Ready

Lie on your side.
Your bottom arm is extended
straight up from your shoulder.
Your elbow is bent and
your hand supports your lifted head.
Place your top arm in front of you,
with your hand flat on the mat for support.
Shoulders are down.
Extend your legs straight down from your hips.
Hips are "stacked" on top of one another.
The powerhouse is pulled in, keeping your lower back long and your chest lifted.
Bring both legs, glued together,
up and forward about 8–12 inches,
so you have an angle in your body.
From the waist up, you're perfectly straight.
From the hips down, you're at an angle.

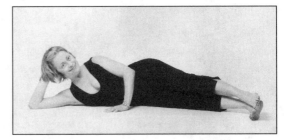

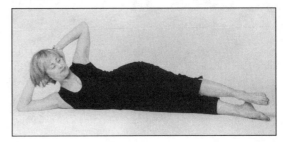

For more advanced levels, place both hands behind your head.

Action

Lift up your top leg
so that it is even with your top hip.
Your ankle is relaxed.
Bring the leg forward as far as you
comfortably can and pulse twice—1, 2.
Think of your leg lengthening, like an arrow
coming out of your hip socket.
Keeping the torso fixed,
bring your top leg down past your bottom leg
and pulse twice to the back—1, 2.
The powerhouse moves the leg.

Repeat 10 times.

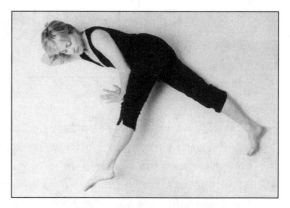

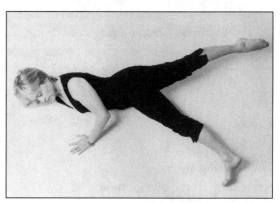

Bicycle Front/Back

Ready

Remain on your side
with your head propped up by your arm.
Bring your top leg straight out in front of
you so that your foot is adjacent to your
belly button.
Bend your knee without moving the thigh,
keeping your knee hip-level.

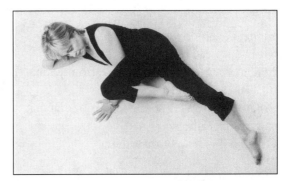

Action

Take your heel toward your buttocks,
shifting that shape to the back,
and then stretch your leg to the back.
Bring your leg straight front.
Repeat 3 times.

Now reverse the direction and
repeat 3 more times.

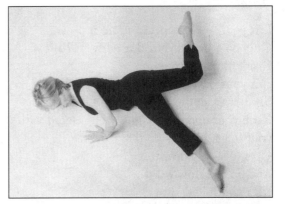

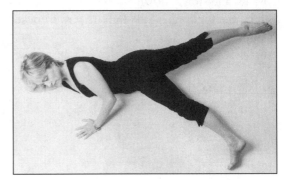

Leg Lifts

Ready

Remain lying on your side
with your head propped up.
Extend your legs straight down from your
hips and at an angle.
Rotate your top leg so the kneecap is facing
toward the ceiling.
One hip is on top of the other.

Action

Lift your top leg up and straight down.
Only go as far as your flexibility will allow.
Don't force anything.
Lift your leg up and bring it down slowly.
Try not to let the upper hip roll back.
Keep your upper hip right in alignment with
your lower hip.
Up and slowly down.
And up and slowly down.
It's a controlled kick.
And up and slowly down.
Again, the torso stays still and the powerhouse
is pulled in.
Ankles are relaxed.

Repeat 10 times.

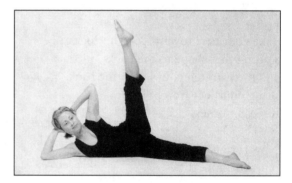

NOTE: This photo demonstrates advanced
arm positioning. If you cannot keep your
torso still with your arms in this position,
simply place your top hand on the mat in
front of you to maintain your balance.

Small Leg Circles

Ready

End the last exercise with your leg extended
or in the "down" position.
Lift your leg until it is even with your hip.
Think of the leg as an arrow
coming out of your hip socket.

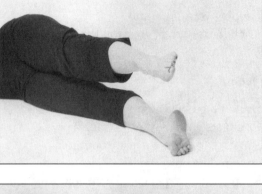

Action

Moving from your hip,
draw a cantaloupe-sized circle with your leg.
Try not to make a circle from your knee or
from your ankle.
Reverse.
Keep the knee and ankle straight.
Keep your powerhouse pulled in.
Do 10 circles in each direction.

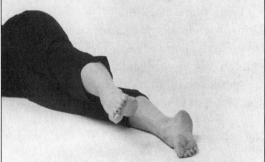

Large Circles

Ready

Keeping your torso still,
reach forward with your top leg.

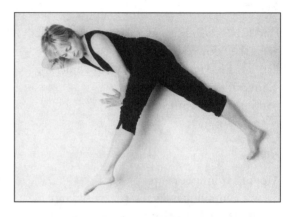

Action

Draw a big circle with your toes.
Completely isolate your top leg.
You have to guide the leg from the hip
by using the powerhouse.
Keep your hips quiet, and your lower leg still.
Pull your powerhouse in.
Don't let your torso waver back and forth.
If you're at a more advanced level on these,
you can pick up the hand that's on the floor
and put it behind your other ear.
Use your powerhouse for control.

Reverse and repeat 5 times.

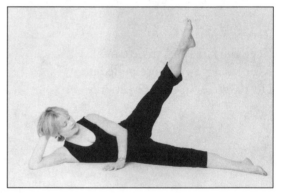

Hot Potato

Ready

Release the top leg down.

Action

Pick up your top leg, and bring it
about 6 inches in front of the bottom leg and
tap your big toe on the floor twice.
Making a half-circle arc, bring your leg
6 inches in back of the bottom leg and tap
your big toe on the floor twice.
You have just completed a repetition.

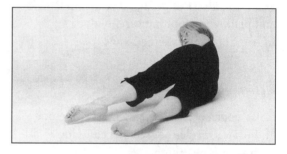

Moving the top leg only slightly higher than
the hip, bring it back in front, and tap twice.

Bring it behind the bottom leg and tap twice.

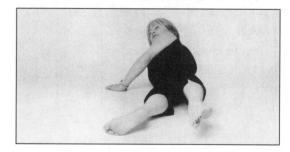

Add some more dynamics to it.

Move the leg to the tempo of
"God Bless America."

Really move it.

Don't forget to breathe.
That's why it's called Hot Potato.

Do 10 repetitions.

Circling the Inner Thighs

Ready

From the Hot Potato, bend your top leg, and place your foot flat on the mat in front of your extended knee.

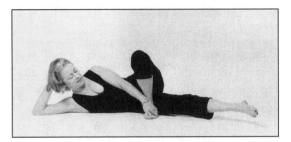

Action

Raise your bottom leg 2 inches off the mat and draw a circle the size of a cantelope with your inner thigh.

Complete 5 clockwise circles and 5 counter-clockwise circles.

Leg Beats

Ready

Both legs are in an angled position.
Glue your legs together.
Using the powerhouse,
lift both legs up 8–10 inches,
or as high as you comfortably can.

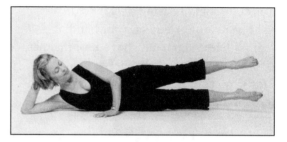

Action

Release your bottom leg down to the mat.
Bring it back up to meet your top leg.
Accent the "up" motion.
The movement should be vigorous.
Repeat 10 times
without resting your bottom leg.

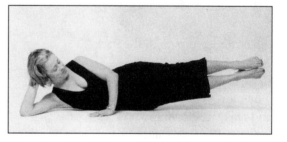

Scissors

Ready

You still should be lying on your side with
your head propped up on your hand.
Lift both legs about 6 inches above the mat,
or as far as you comfortably can.
Don't roll your hips to the back; stack your
legs on top of one another.

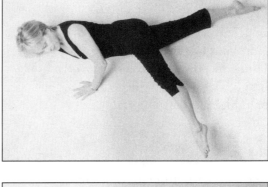

Action

Move one leg to the front as
the other leg moves to the back.
Now switch.
Just like a pair of scissors.
The movement is fluid and balanced,
and emanates from the powerhouse.
Pick up the tempo and
make the movement bigger.
Give yourself some space between the ankles.
Your powerhouse should be pushing in
toward the spine.

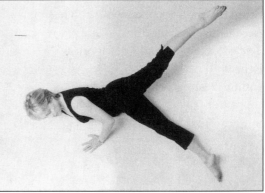

Repeat 10 times.

**NOW ROLL OVER AND
REPEAT THIS SERIES ON YOUR OTHER SIDE.**

Teaser #1

If you have a bad lower back, I do not recommend this exercise.
In addition to flattening your tummy, you should also feel your spine
lengthen. To achieve this, you want to feel like someone is pulling your torso
away from your hips as you roll down.

Prep

Lie flat on your back,
keeping your spine long against the floor
and your belly button toward the spine.
Relax your shoulders and
keep your arms by your side,
palms against the mat.
Reach your arms over your head and stretch.

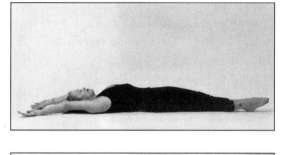

Action

Raise your legs to a 45-degree angle.
As you inhale
reach your arms up toward the ceiling.
As your arms
become perpendicular to the ceiling,
use your powerhouse
to lift your head and shoulders off the mat.
Pull your shoulders down.
Come up until
you are balanced on your "sit-bones"
in a "V"-shape position.

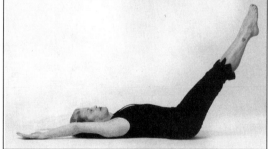

Keeping your legs fixed,
slowly roll down vertebra by vertebra.
Use the powerhouse
to control the movement.
And again.
Don't stop the movement of your arms.
Continue to reach.
The reach and the powerhouse pull you up.
Come to a point of balance.
Pull the abdominals in toward the lower back
and exhale as you
roll down vertebra by vertebra.
Once more.
Arms come up first.
Chin to your chest.
Come to a point of balance and
roll down slowly through the vertebrae,
breathing as you go.
Relax.
Hug your knees gently to your chest.

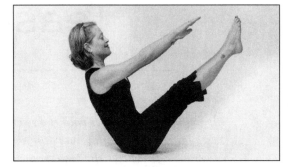

Teaser #2

Again, if you have a bad back, I do not recommend this exercise. As you complete this exercise, you should be feeling it in your abdominal muscles. As you become more advanced, you can lower your legs closer and closer to the mat.

Ready

Lie flat on your back, keeping
your legs at a 45-degree angle.
Your arms extend and relax straight up above
your shoulders with palms facing the ceiling.
Pull your shoulders down.

Action

Inhale without arching the lower back.
Slowly reach your arms toward your feet until
you have come to a point of balance on top of
your "sit-bones," and your arms and legs are
reaching out along parallel lines.
Pull the powerhouse into your lower spine.
Lower your legs down, then bring them back
up 3 times.

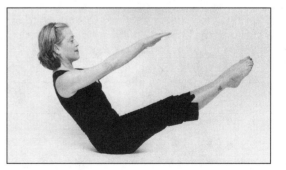

Exhale as you lower yourself down slowly.
Keep reaching your arms toward your feet,
so that you are rolling down one vertebra at a
time and maintaining the curve in your back.
Pull your torso away from your hips.
Pull the powerhouse into your spine as you
release the upper back into the mat.
Arms reach above the head and stretch long.

Repeat 3–5 times.

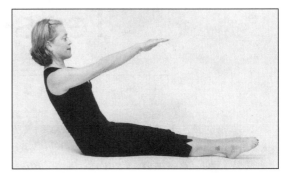

Teaser #3

If you are feeling confident, and have mastered Teaser #2, this advanced exercise will really work the abdominal muscles. Think of yourself folding and unfolding like an oriental fan, or like a clothespin. Use your hip socket or the fold of the leg as a hinge.

Ready

Lie flat on your back.
Legs are long against the mat.
Your arms should be stretched above your
shoulders, keeping them long against the mat.
Using the connection of the powerhouse,
feel energized from the tips of your fingers
down through the toes.

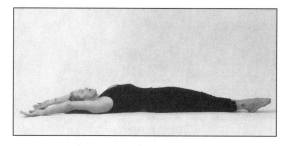

Action

Inhale as you glue your legs together;
from the powerhouse
reach your arms and lift your legs
simultaneously until you come to a point of
balance on top of your "sit-bones."
You are now in a "V" position,
with your arms and legs reaching just past
your ears on parallel lines.

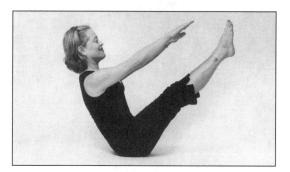

Exhale as you
use the powerhouse to
simultaneously lower your legs
and roll down through your back.
Continue holding your arms by your ears
until you are in a prone position on the mat.

Repeat 3–5 times.

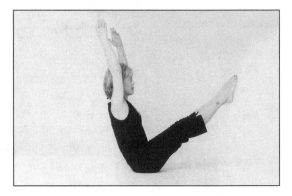

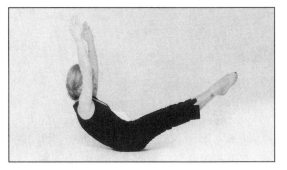

Single Leg Teaser

This is the most advanced Teaser exercise. It is designed to really work all of the abdominal musculature and to strengthen the powerhouse.

Ready

Lie flat on your back,
with your arms on the mat above your head.
Pull the powerhouse into your lower spine.
The spine is now long, your shoulders and
neck are relaxed. Your chest is lifted.
Draw your right foot in toward your buttocks,
with your kneecap pointing toward the ceiling,
and place your right foot flat against the mat.

Action

Extend your left leg straight out from your
hip socket, and lift it toward the ceiling until
it is at a 45-degree angle and the knees are
touching.
Inhale as you
bring your arms straight back,
without lifting up your shoulders.
Sweep your arms up and reach your arms
parallel to your right thigh.
Pull in your powerhouse and come up into a
"V"-shaped Teaser position.
Take your arms up by your ears,
pull your belly button into your lower spine,
and exhale as you
pull your pelvis underneath you and slowly
roll down, keeping your arms by your ears as
long as you can.

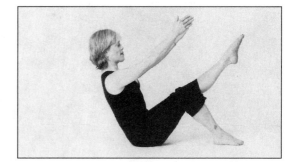

Come back up.
When you reach the "V" position,
twist your body over the bent knee,
twist back to the center,
stretch your arms up toward the ceiling,
and slowly roll down. Now you have
completed one set.

Do 2 sets on each side.

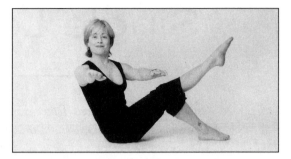

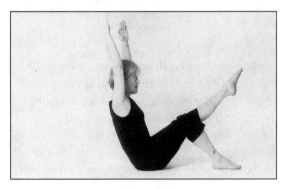

Hip Circles

This exercise is like a sitting corkscrew. The more advanced you are, the larger the circle. At a very advanced level, you would sweep your legs past each ear as you circle. Again, it does not matter how high or how far you go, you are only working on controlling the movement with the powerhouse. I do not recommend this exercise if you have a bad back.

Transition

After the last teaser,
roll up one more time into
the check-mark position.
Circle your arms behind you,
and place your palms on the mat
with your fingers pointing away from you.

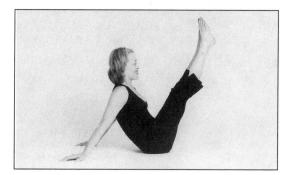

Ready

With your torso now at a 45-degree angle,
lift your legs as high as you comfortably can.
Tweeze your ribs together,
and pull the powerhouse in.
Glue your legs together, and
glue your buttocks to the floor.

Action

Inhale as you
draw your legs to your left.
Exhale as you circle your legs,
sweeping them down toward the mat,
and then swing them up until
you are in the check-mark position (center).

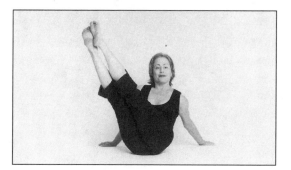

Now reverse the action.
Try not to let your lower back arch.
Draw down, around, up, and center.
This is a very controlled movement,
and it should not be done quickly.
Keep your arms as straight as you can.
The abdominal muscles are drawn in
and the legs are controlled.
Do not let those legs come apart or bend.
Repeat 3–5 times.

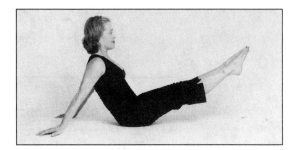

Can-Can

This exercise is a great release for the back after you do Hip Circles. It is great for slimming and creating definition in your waistline. It is also really good for lengthening your thighs and hamstrings, and for releasing or stretching the lower back muscles.

Ready

After Hip-Circles,
remain leaning on your hands,
with your torso inclined at a 45-degree angle.
Lengthen your legs,
extending them straight out from your hips,
and bend your knees in toward you.
Place your toes on the floor and
bring your knees as close to you as you can.
Don't let your legs or your ankles separate.

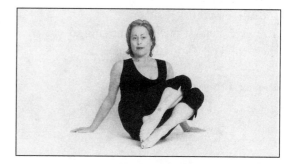

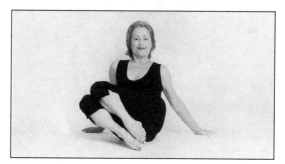

Action

Let your legs fall to the right side
so that you are mainly on your right hip.
Bring them back through center
and let them fall to your left side.
Move back through center to the right.
Keep your thighs where they are, and pull
the powerhouse in to straighten your legs.
Bend your knees back again
without moving your thighs.
This is a "set."

Now repeat this motion,
starting on your left side.
You may pick up the pace, moving to
the tempo of "God Bless America."

Repeat 5 times.

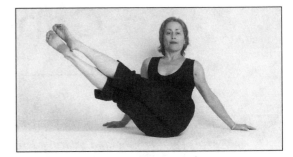

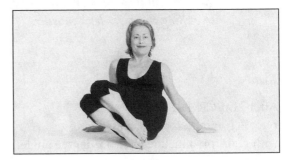

Kneeling Side Kicks

Transition

From the Can-Can,
bring your right knee underneath you,
and then the left.
Kneel and come up to center.
Push your pelvis forward slightly.
Lengthen your lower back.
Stretch out your sides a little before you begin.
Standing straight up on your knees,
drop your right hand toward the mat and
feel the stretch in your left ribs.
Come back to center.
Drop your left hand toward the mat and
feel the stretch in your right ribs.

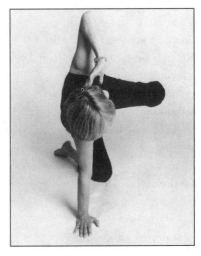

Ready

Lean to your right.
Let your right hand keep you from falling.
The right hand is now directly under your
shoulder.
Your right hip is directly over your right knee.
Extend your left leg to the side so it is parallel
with the mat.
Your head stays in the middle of your
shoulder blades.
Place your left hand behind your head,
pulling the elbow so it makes a straight line
with your right arm.

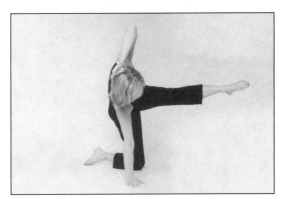

Action

Inhale as you tweeze the buttocks together,
and tighten the muscles in your powerhouse.
Exhale and sweep your leg gently forward.
Keep your leg level,
like it is moving through a tunnel,
until it is in front of your hip
at a right angle with your body.
Inhale as you take your leg back—
not too far if you have a tight back.
Keep it level.
Try this slowly 2 more times.
Now swing your leg front and back.
Maintain the same amount of control and
keep your leg on an even level.

Repeat 5 times.

Come back to center
and repeat on the other side.

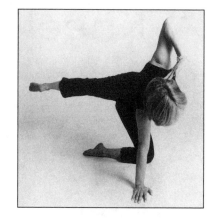

The Mermaid

This exercise is designed to open up your rib cage and stretch your waist.

Transition

From the Kneeling Side Kicks,
bring your left hip down to the mat
so that you are sitting on your left hip,
with your knees bent and facing forward
(right knee on top of the left, right foot on
top of the left).

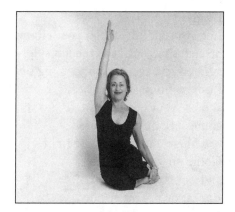

Ready

Your right hand
should hold the right ankle for balance.
Stretch your left arm
straight up above your shoulder.
There should be a straight line between
your left hip and left hand.
Pull the powerhouse in, and continue to
lengthen along your entire left side.

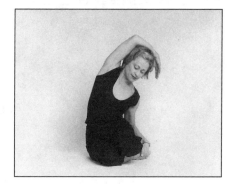

Action

Let your left arm fall over your head,
and reach your body toward the right side.
Feel the stretch in your left ribs.
Extend your left arm straight up again.
Pull your lats down. Your neck is long.
Reach your left hand down to the mat,
fingers pointing away from you.
Stretch the right arm up and over your head,
with your fingertips pointed away from you.
Pull your powerhouse into your spine.
Lengthen.
Lean to your left and let your elbow bend.
Stretch straight out to the left side,
as far as you can without coming off the mat.
Push up from your forearm
and use your powerhouse to
come back through center,
reaching your torso to the right.
Come up onto your knees
and sit on your right hip.
Repeat on the other side.
Repeat this exercise 2 more times.

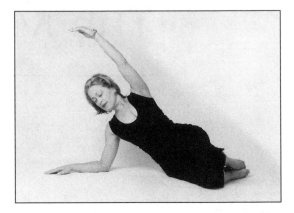

Scissors

In this exercise, you will be moving your legs in opposition. Your legs should act as counterbalances for one another. It does not matter how far you move your legs. You are working on your balance and controlling the movement. The more advanced you are, the greater the range of motion. Only go as far as you comfortably can. Again, I would not recommend this exercise for people with bad necks or bad backs.

Ready

Lie flat on your back, with your neck long.
Pull your shoulders down.
Your legs should be extended straight out from your hips.
Arms are against your sides, with the palms against the mat.

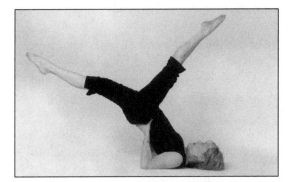

Action

Lift both legs overhead,
bringing them parallel to the floor.
Place your hands underneath your hips,
with your elbows against the mat.
Separate your legs like scissors.
Stay within the frame of your hips.
Each leg moves to counterbalance the other.
One leg moves toward your face,
as your other leg reaches toward the floor.
The focus is downward with the reaching leg.
Control comes from the powerhouse.
Move your legs as far as flexibility allows.
With a brisk tempo, switch legs.
Repeat 4 times.

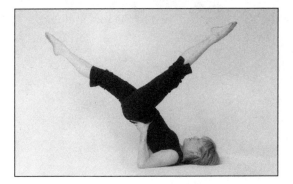

Bicycle

Generally, you should not do this exercise if you have a bad neck. If this exercise hurts your neck or lower back, don't do it.

Action

From the Scissors, use the powerhouse to
bring your knees into your chest.
Point your legs backward
to where the ceiling and the wall meet.
From this position, reach your left leg as close
to the floor as you can, bend your knee and
draw your leg back up in a bicycle motion.

Turn the bicycle wheel 4 times in one
direction, and then reverse the rotation of the
wheel 4 times.

Relax your back down to the mat and take a
few deep breaths.

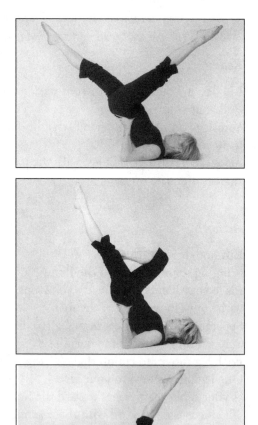

Shoulder Bridge

This exercise provides a wonderful stretch for your hamstrings and really works your abdominal muscles. I do not recommend this exercise if you have a bad lower back, a bad neck, tennis elbow, or carpal tunnel syndrome.

Ready

Lie flat on your back.
Bend your knees.
Your feet should be flat on the mat directly under your knees.
Your knees should be hip-width apart.
Feel your whole spine against the mat.
Your ribs should be relaxed,
and your neck long.
Pull your shoulders down.
Your weight is now on
your elbows and your shoulders.
To create some length in your hip area,
pull in the powerhouse as you
tweeze both your pelvis and your buttocks.

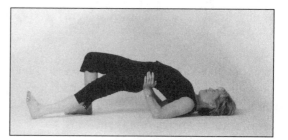

Action

Scoop your pelvis up and
bring yourself up vertebra by vertebra.
Continue to curl up until only
your shoulder blades are touching the mat.
Bend your elbows and
put your hands underneath your hips,
so that the fingers are facing up and
the elbows are slightly open,
away from your torso.
Your knees
should be almost even with your hips.
Pull your ribs in as much as you can,
and keep your neck long.
Extend your right leg out straight,
without making any adjustments in your hip.
Actually reach your foot down to the floor,
and bending your knee, use the foot like a
paintbrush to "paint" the floor.
Bring your knee toward you
and then stretch your leg straight up
so that it is pointed toward the ceiling.
Bring your leg straight down,
using your foot to paint the ceiling and wall.

Repeat 4 times for each leg.

When you are finished, plant your feet, then
slowly release your arms and slowly pull your
rib cage in. Roll down one vertebra at a time,
"unscooping" your pelvis for the last four
vertebrae until your back is completely
against the mat.

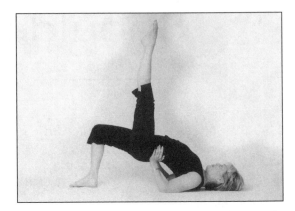

Leg Pull Down

As you lift your leg, you will be pushing your heel back. As your leg comes back down, you will be coming up on the ball of your foot. This will stretch your Achilles tendon and your calf muscles.

Ready

Come to a push-up position,
keeping your feet hip-width apart,
heels over your toes.
Hands are underneath your shoulders.
Fingertips are facing forward.
Your body should be flat like a board.
Look straight down, keep your neck long.
Pull your powerhouse tightly into your spine.
Tweeze the buttocks tightly.

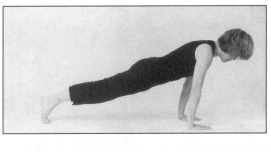

Action

Push your right heel back as you lift your
left leg as high as you comfortably can.
Come back on the ball of your foot,
heel over toes,
as you bring the leg down.
The torso remains fixed,
and the buttocks stay tight.
Repeat as you lift your right leg.
Do 3 sets.

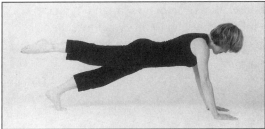

Leg Pull Up

This is a great exercise for your abdominal muscles as well as your triceps. You don't want your pelvis to sink as the leg raises up, and you don't want the hips to shift. You can keep your hips square by pulling the powerhouse in and tweezing your buttocks tightly.

Transition

Circle your left arm around
as you swing your body over.
Your buttocks are now facing downward.

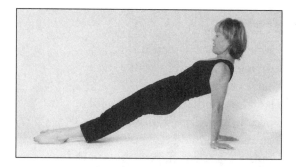

Ready

Both hands are underneath your shoulders,
fingers are facing out.
Tweeze your buttocks in toward the powerhouse and lift them up as high as you can.
Pull the powerhouse in even more, and
keep the body flat. You are now in the
opposite position of a push-up.
Glue the legs together and rest on your heels.

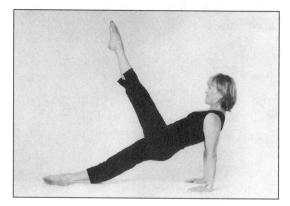

Action

Inhale and raise your right leg
upward and toward you.
It doesn't have to be high.
It's just for control and strength.
Pull your shoulders down.
Your neck should be long and relaxed.
Exhale as you bring your leg down.
Lift your pelvis up higher as you come down.
Continue to breathe evenly as
you lift your leg up and down.
Repeat 3 times on each side.

Boomerang

This is a really great stretch for your upper back and scapula. The motion of your arms will really loosen that area up. You will be primarily focused on your powerhouse and maintaining your balance. The entire body is involved in moving over and back from a center point. The contraction of the powerhouse initiates the rolling back. Your hip, the point where your leg folds into the pelvis, is operating like the hinge of a clothespin. This hinge helps to control the movement of the legs.

Ready

Sit upright, balancing
on top of your "sit-bones."
Your legs extend out from your hip sockets.
Cross your right ankle over the left.

Arms are down, palms are flat against the mat.
Pull down your shoulders, and relax your ribs,
keeping your torso long.

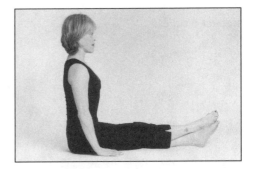

Action

Inhale as you
pull the powerhouse into your spine,
so you have a nice "C" curve in your back.
As you roll back,
your legs are lifted off the mat.
As you bring your legs over your head,
switch positions with your ankles
(left ankle on top of the right ankle).
Roll down slowly—vertebra by vertebra.

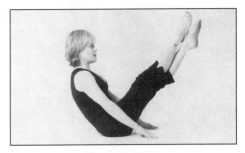

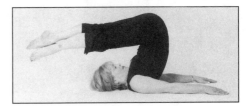

Roll back up with control and temporarily
hold the position when your torso reaches a
45-degree angle or "Teaser position."
Pull the powerhouse in.
Exhale as you hold your balance,
sweep your arms around to the back,
clasp your hands behind your lower back,
and pull to stretch open the shoulders as
the legs are lowered down.
As soon as your legs touch the floor,
Pull your powerhouse in toward your spine.
Curve your upper body over the legs,
reaching your arms up and over your head.
Lengthen your neck and
reach your fingers toward your feet.

Repeat 3 times.

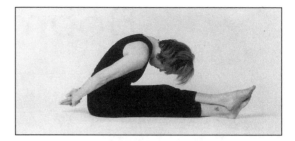

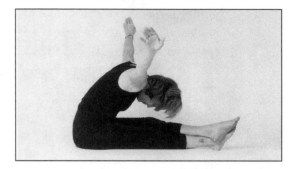

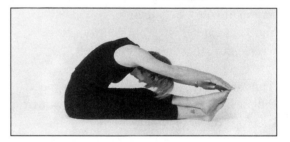

The Seal

The Seal is a cool-down exercise that relaxes your spine, actually massaging it as you're rolling back and forth. It works on your abdominals for balance and is also a test for your coordination. This entire exercise is really guided by the powerhouse. You will be pushing the powerhouse into your spine so that you maintain a nice curve in your back.

Ready

Begin this exercise sitting up tall
with your knees bent, open, and relaxed.
The soles of your feet should be together.
Slide your hands underneath your ankles.
Place your elbows
to the inside of the bent knees, causing
your back to be bent in a nice "C" curve.

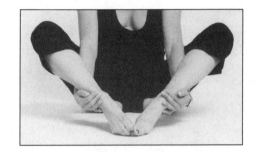

Action

Inhale as you
bring the powerhouse into the spine,
and gently roll back.
Hold the movement as you
balance on top of your shoulders,
tapping your heels together 3 times.
As you exhale,
use the powerhouse to roll back up.
(Don't let your feet touch the mat.)
Balance on top of your "sit-bones" and
tap your heels together 3 times.

Repeat 6 times.

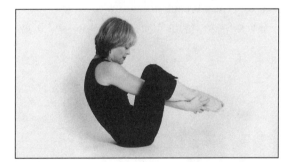

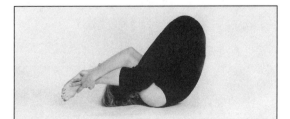

Push-Ups

With this exercise, you can clearly see the lineage of eastern disciplines in Pilates's work. This particular exercise is based on yoga's "Solar Salutation." As you become more advanced in this work, when you reach the point of actually doing the push-up, you can put one ankle behind the other and keep that leg extended throughout the exercise.

Ready

Stand tall at the end of the mat.

Action

Drop your head gently, and let the
weight of your head pull your body down,
rolling down vertebra by vertebra,
keeping the rib cage pulled in.
If you can touch your toes, great. If not, it's okay.

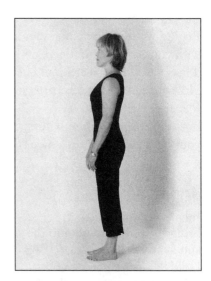

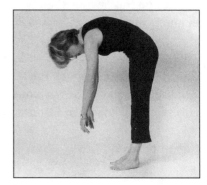

Walk your hands out on the mat.
Make an "A" with your body.
Use the powerhouse to guide the weight
of your body
toward your hands until your entire body is
flat, in a push-up position.
Inhale as you
ease your body down toward the mat,
and exhale as you push up—
keeping the entire body as straight as a board.
Do 5 push-ups.

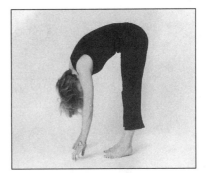

Walk your hands back toward the feet,
pushing your heels down into the mat.
Pull the powerhouse in, and
curl your pelvis underneath you.
Roll up slowly
as you stack one vertebra on top of the other.
Let your powerhouse guide the movement.
Your head is the last to come up.
Take your arms up in the air
and lift your sternum toward the ceiling.

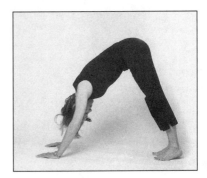

Don't arch the lower back—just the upper back.
Look toward the ceiling
without collapsing your neck.
Now, let your arms fall to your sides,
and drop your head down.

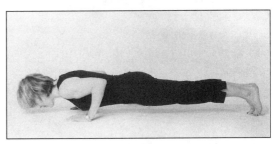

Repeat 3 times.

Total Butt Workout

This is not a Pilates exercise, but one of my own. My clients love what this does for their buttocks.

Ready

Lie on your back with your
feet against the wall.
Your legs should be at a 45-degree angle.
Put a ball between your knees and squeeze.
Squeeze for 10 counts.
Squeeze again.
Tweeze your buttocks together.
Come back to neutral.
Scoot yourself forward.
Your legs are now against the wall at a
right angle.

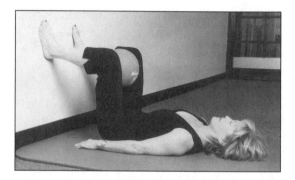

Action

Tweeze your buttocks and scoop your hips up.
Your pelvis will act like an ice-cream scooper.
Stomach in and scoop up.
Scoop your pelvis up toward the ceiling.
Take your pelvis as high as you can without
arching the back.
Release down,
vertebra by vertebra.
Repeat 10 times.
Scoop your pelvis toward the ceiling
and stay there.

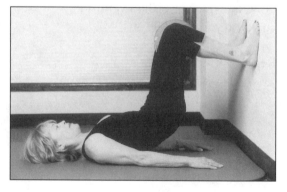

Pulse your pelvis upward toward the ceiling.
Your range of motion should be no more than
3 inches. Engage your abdominal muscles for
each pulse.
Keep the tweeze in your buttocks.
Continue pulsing at least 50 times.
Come back down to neutral,
vertebra by vertebra.

Closing

Now to finish up.
Scoot your butt to the wall
and stretch your legs straight up.
Keep your legs together.
Put a pillow under your head if you need to.
Stay in this position for a few minutes and
take some deep breaths.
Take a deep breath in through your nose
and out through your mouth.
Wring those lungs out.
Make a connection with your breath
and to the abdominal muscles.
Inhale through the nose.
Exhale through the mouth.
One more time.

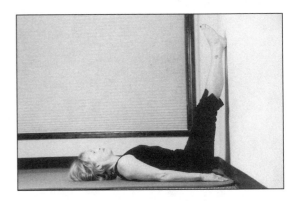

Injuries and Injury Prevention

"Not only do I credit my professional longevity to the preventative attributes of Pilates, but I was able to rehabilitate my body back from a very severe injury."

—Mari Winsor

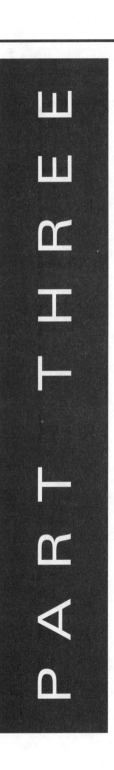

PART THREE

Defying Defeat

CHAPTER 6

*"Mari Winsor has changed my posture
and helped my back immeasurably
with Pilates exercise."*
—DUSTIN HOFFMAN

*"Pilates has healed my hamstring,
increased my flexibility and overall strength."*
—JASMINE GUY

*"Doing Pilates with Mari Winsor every night
during the shooting of* Lethal Weapon IV *was
instrumental in keeping me strong and
physically fit for the film."*
—DANNY GLOVER

Healing Injuries and Injury Prevention:
What Would Your Doctor Say?

When you are attempting to recover from an injury or have chronic pain, it is *essential* that you check with your doctor. It is quite possible that your doctor doesn't actually know what Pilates is, so bring this book in on your next doctor's visit so he or she can assess these exercises, and so that *you* can be absolutely certain that this workout will not be harmful to your recovery in any way. If your injury stems from a bone or cartilage problem, I would seek not only the counsel of your doctor, but that of a physical therapist as well, since many physical therapists incorporate Pilates into rehabilitation programs. Chances are, both doctors and physical therapists will say this is exactly what you should be doing on a daily basis. If you are experiencing any pain and/or chronic pain that is muscular in nature, this exercise regimen will definitely be for you. It may be just the "miracle" that you are seeking.

The great majority of people who suffer from chronic pain do not consult a doctor, because they don't think their pain is significant enough, or bothersome enough, to seek professional help. But the nagging pain is often a symptom of an overall injury condition. Your body may be trying to tell you something important, and my advice is not to ignore that "voice." Do yourself a favor. If you have chronic pain, get a professional opinion.

Many people gravitate toward Pilates as a regular form of rehabilitation to heal an injury. Once they experience the dramatic benefits of this regimen, Pilates becomes a lifestyle. This exercise routine is fantastic for aiding in recovery from and the prevention of injuries. Although the focus of this chapter is on injuries, we will also be discussing the basic principles of this method of body conditioning. If you have picked up this book because you are looking to alleviate chronic pain, are in physical therapy or rehabilitation for an injury, or would like to do as much as you possibly can to avoid injury, you picked up the right book.

I can personally attest to the benefits of Pilates. I was a trained professional dancer, performing on video and film and on stage.

Like athletes, dancers have a finite career. Because dancing is so physically rigorous, by the time you are approaching your late twenties, it may be time to start looking for a new career. By using this method of body conditioning, I was able to dance professionally until I was well into my forties. I mention this only so that you can more fully understand how many pulled muscles, how many injuries, and how much pain I had to work through without letting on that I may not have been feeling my best. These injuries can be serious for someone who moves for a living. When athletes play despite their injuries, that decision oftentimes will be career-threatening. Pilates, however, enabled me to perform at high levels over a very long career, and stay strong as I grew older. Pilates helped me attain higher levels of performance, cope with the rigorous physical regimen, eliminate the potential for career-ending injuries, and remain in peak physical condition.

Not only do I credit my professional longevity to the preventative attributes of Pilates, but I was also able to rehabilitate my body back from a very severe injury. I was riding on the back of a friend's motorcycle after attending my twentieth high school reunion in rural Michigan. It was after midnight and the roads were deserted. I have no recollection of the accident, but when I came to, I was looking into the eyes of a dead deer. Then the pain hit me. I couldn't breathe because my lung was punctured and because so many of my ribs were broken. In the emergency room, I was told that in addition to the injuries to my lung and ribs, I had also severely bruised my heart. I had broken some fingers and my collarbone. The worst of it, however, was that my hips had literally exploded. Apparently I had landed directly on my hip and shoulder during the fall.

After a few days in the hospital, the doctors warned me that I was not going to be moving easily for at least a year. Friends who came to visit me couldn't believe that I had actually lived through the accident. My appearance was so disconcerting that some of them were actually frightened by the sight of me. The pain was horrendous. And I literally could not move. I couldn't get up to go to the bathroom . . . nothing. After two weeks in the hospital, the doctors told me that dance would never come easy to me again. I responded that they didn't know me and had no way to judge my resolve, and I tried to demonstrate with my limited capacity what a fighter I was. Their response was a condescending and doubtful "Well, maybe in time."

After my broken bones mended, I started doing the routine that you'll find in this book. The first time I attempted it, I was really suffering, but it wasn't from the pain. Although the pain was excruciating, my desire to move again had kind of anesthetized me. I was despondent because I couldn't move in the way I had just weeks before. You can never really know what a joyous miracle movement is until that ability is taken away from you. The things that I had once done so effortlessly and had taken for granted were just a memory. I gathered all the resolve I could muster and swore to myself that I wouldn't stop until I had not only met my former performance level but had surpassed it. Each day I went a little further. Each day I pushed myself a little harder. Two months later I was dancing again.

If you have pain, I can honestly say that I understand. With compassion, I offer you this advice: Do as much as you can to work with your pain. If your doctor says you have scar tissue around an old injury, an old break, the singularly most important thing that you can do is break apart that scar tissue. One of the only ways to do that is to stretch. Stretch it out. It may be painful, but in most cases you can work through the pain. In the case of a pulled muscle, I urge you to work extremely slowly. Work up to the pain. In other words, work until you can feel that it is uncomfortable. Try to go a little bit further each day. For instance, if you have an injured hamstring, keep the rest of your body conditioned and strong and take the time to stretch your lower back thoroughly. You will find that you can bend over a little bit further each day. Even if it is only a quarter of an inch—that is progress. In eight days it will be two inches. In a month? You decide. That kind of growth becomes exciting and addictive. It gives you a sense of accomplishment. Most important, it gives you a sense of control. When we are injured, we lose that sense of control that we have over our bodies. More than the movement that we have lost or that is now restricted, what we truly mourn is the loss of our sense of control. Working diligently and concertedly wrests the control over our bodies back from the fates that took it from us. To me, desire is the most important aspect of the healing process.

Put simply, you must make up your mind that you cannot be defeated. When we have an injury that prevents us from doing what we normally do or what we want to do, we feel defeated, debilitated, and exhausted, mentally and physically. If you give in to those feelings, you give in to defeat. It's like shaking your fist at the sky and shouting at the top of your lungs, "Why me? I'm a good person. Why did this happen to me?" You *cannot* and *must not* let your pain defeat you. When you can work through your pain, you *can* come out on the other side. You can be as good, or even better than you were before. That is a victory of the highest order. What occurs when you achieve these kinds of victories translates positively into the rest of your life in thousands of ways. If you can go through something like that and come out victorious, what can stop you from achieving business and family goals? What can possibly stop you from achieving your dreams? Defy defeat!

Chronic Pain

The Pilates method of body conditioning is often a perfect remedy for healing or diminishing chronic pain. In fact, most doctors and physical therapists who are familiar with this method of conditioning will recommend it to their patients. The reasons for this are quite simple: When you commit yourself to this form of exercise, you are strengthening muscle groups that have been weakened or atrophied. You are developing smaller muscle groups that support larger muscles. You create a balance of strength in musculature and increase overall circulation, thereby bringing more oxygen into the muscles. Most important, this exercise is scientifically designed to eliminate or drastically diminish the risk of re-injuring or exacerbating the problem or the area from which the pain emanates.

Most of you who suffer from chronic pain know only that you have it, but are not sure where to turn for a solution. Chronic pain can be attributed to several possible causes: age, respiratory problems, the lasting effects of a previous injury, a weakness of musculature that does not allow it to support the body's posture properly, stress, or a lifestyle that fosters the pain.

Age

Right up front, let's first dismiss a myth about age. You are never too old to be active. My mentor is in her seventies and still performs this routine and teaches it.

Pilates will not jar or harm the body in any way if it is performed correctly. In fact, performing this particular exercise routine can offset some of the physical weakness, muscular atrophy, balance, and osteoporosis issues that face the aging. Aside from the physical benefits, this routine will improve your circulation, and you will feel an improved sense of mental clarity. Because you will have to focus and to remember which exercise comes next, you may find that Pilates helps you to hone your memory. As you practice Pilates, you will increase your strength and flexibility, and also receive a wealth of secondary mental benefits that will give you an overall sense of well-being. The most difficult thing about aging is that we reach the point where we begin to question ourselves. After a couple of falls, or a few bouts of bad health, we begin not to trust ourselves. But, each time you practice this routine, you will feel a little bit more confident in your movement. You will trust your balance a little bit more and feel infinitely more invigorated afterward.

Respiratory Problems

The most basic and important human bodily function is breathing. And breathing is a key aspect of the Pilates method of body conditioning. As you learn to perform this routine you will also learn to link breath with movement so that you can nourish your musculature with oxygen. Even if you are fortunate enough to not have a respiratory problem, breathing is a very important area of focus both in nourishing the body and easing the mind. Because breathing is essential to living, when we have difficulty with it, the ramifications are numerous. Ailments such as asthma and emphysema affect breathing more than any other respiratory disease or disorder. If we can offset the effects of these diseases, we can certainly create at least a partial solution to most respiratory concerns.

When asthmatics have an attack, their bronchial tubes start to close up and their bodies get very tense. This is totally understandable; the person's life is becoming increasingly threatened as he or she fights harder and harder to breathe. The very intensity of the struggle to breathe forces the muscles to contract around the lungs and make the bronchial tubes even smaller. When you suffer an asthma attack, it's important to say to yourself, "Okay, try to relax. Try to relax your muscles." If you should ever have an attack while performing this routine or any other activity, you *must* stop exercising. However, if you are experiencing only minor breathing difficulty when performing this routine, instead of trying to breathe normally, I want you to stay with your movements and then concentrate on your breath, making certain to fully exhale. Get all the air out. When we have asthma, we gasp and wheeze because we're fighting to get the air in, and we are not pushing enough air out. As a result, our breath is strained and very shallow as we try to gasp in as much air as we can. But we need to create more room in our lungs for the air we are about to take in. Expel all of that contaminated air inside of you and breathe in fresh air to rejuvenate the body.

Joseph Pilates had terrible asthma, as do I. I fully understand the repercussions that breathing problems have throughout the body. Over time it can dramatically affect our posture and our quality of life in general. Based on the sheer number of people who suffer from this particular ailment, I have compiled a series of exercises just for lending some comfort to your breathing. I have found that it has helped me immensely over the years. Knock on wood, I have been able to alleviate my wheezing, and I have not had a major attack or flare-up. Although I still carry around my inhaler, I have not had to use it for a very long time.

Previous Injuries

Physical injuries can also severely alter the way we move and hold ourselves. Even after our bones have mended and the scars have faded, the effects of these injuries sometimes stay with us for the rest of our lives. When the wounds heal, we are left with scar tissue or other lasting physical reminders of the injury. Earlier in this chapter, I shared with you the importance of stretching to break up scar tissue in order to free the body for an increased range of motion. Through the Pilates method of body conditioning, I have helped people from all walks of life—dancers, actors, athletes, businesspeople, and housewives—erase the remnants of previous injuries that eventually could have become disabling.

As a trainer, I am particularly concerned if clients come to me complaining of chronic pain. If they are under the supervision of a medical practitioner, I like to consult the professional to determine where the basic problem may lie, and then I will find a way to work on those parts of the body. I look at two basic areas. I look at the client's posture, paying careful attention to the way people stand and carry their body. Then I observe their gait, their walk, to see how they move their body. Often, chronic pain reveals its true origin through these important functions. If neither of these reveals the mystery, I try to find out what they do for a living. Perhaps one of the redundant tasks that they perform throughout the day may be contributing to this pain. If that is not the answer, then I look at what they do for activities. Once the problem area is identified, I can design or emphasize certain exercises.

Since I cannot be with you personally, I will ask you to be this careful observer. It is actually more important that you discover and reveal these problems areas yourself. Once you perceive these areas, you can fully understand how important Pilates is for your overall well-being.

Your Posture

Ask yourself: "How is my posture?" First, I want you to examine how you stand. Is your chest collapsed in on itself? Do you cock your head to one side all the time? When you stand and look at yourself in profile, do you jut your neck out? The shoulder area is often the major culprit when we talk about poor posture. Are your shoulders hunched over? Many people throw their shoulders back.

Do you? When you were a kid, you would be slouching at the dinner table. Your mother would tell you to sit up straight. At her command you would throw your shoulders back. However, this can pinch your upper back. Do it once. You see, the weight of your shoulders is going backwards and all that weight must be supported by the lower back instead of the stomach muscles. The entire weight of your torso should be over your hips, so that your hips and your stomach support that very heavy area of the body, keeping it upright and balanced. The body was designed to be in alignment to properly support all its weight. When our posture is not balanced, we aren't in proper alignment. Joseph Pilates said that the spine should be straight like a Greek column. When we are not aligned, the muscles become overburdened from carrying the load that should be displaced over our bone structure. As a result, those muscles will either get tighter from overuse or will atrophy from underuse because they are not holding anything. If you continue to ignore these basic posture-related areas of concern, the chronic pain will spread in an ever-increasing radius.

Your Walk

This isn't a finishing class, but let's now examine how you walk. Do what you normally do, no better and no worse. Just observe in a mirror how you are moving. Do you walk with one leg turned in? Do you walk with one leg turned out? Do you swing your arms too much? Do you drop your head down too low and always look at the ground? Do you carry a baby in one arm all the time? Or a shoulder bag? Are your limbs within the frame of the body? Are they supported, or are they extending over the boundaries of your body? Do you carry most of your weight on your heels? Do you walk toe-ball-heel? Do you hold your stomach in to support your back? Do you lock your knees when you walk? Is your foot underneath the hip? Are your knees soft and not hyperextended? In merely becoming aware of how you walk, you can go to work to correct the problem. You want to be mindful of these things, because moving without proper support of your body can have many far-reaching negative effects. Pilates can correct not only the way you walk but it will also help to keep you within the frame of your body and properly support its weight. You can thus alleviate much of the pain associated with the way you move.

Your Lifestyle

What we do each day—and may not be fully aware of—can also be the root of our chronic pain. What do you do for a living? Could that be a causative factor in this chronic pain? Are you slouching because you sit at a computer all day long and don't stretch? Do you travel a lot and carry a lot of heavy luggage? Do you ride horses all day long? Are you a race-car driver . . . do you feel your upper back is always scrunched? Are you a homemaker, always cooking and reaching? Is that why your shoulders and neck always hurt? Are you a schoolteacher and on your feet all the time? Do your hips and legs always ache? Do you stand all day long on concrete and feel like the arches in your feet are collapsing? Is there anything that you do throughout the day that is repetitive? If you work on an assembly line, you commit the body to do one set of tasks all day long. Is that wearing on your body? What do you do as an activity or for regular exercise? When you go jogging, are you running on uneven sand? Are you running on cement? Are you running on the treadmill? These can all be areas of concern when we have chronic pain.

What we do each and every day is truly a lifestyle issue. Let's say you sit at a computer all day long, and you're hunched over when you come home. All of a sudden your body starts to break down. The slouch leads to back problems . . . the back problems lead to neck problems . . . neck and back problems lead to knee problems. Pretty soon you are not physically willing or able to move in any way, shape, or form. The longer you remain inactive, the worse your ailments get. It's a cycle, a merry-go-round. Once you are part of that, you just resign yourself. It has happened over time without your ever really thinking about it. You don't think how different life would be if your posture was improved. Pilates represents a shift in orientation from a lack of awareness to that of healing the body and preventing injury.

The link between the root cause of your chronic pain and your ability to prevent future injury is a close one. The causes of chronic pain are key in understanding how we injure ourselves. Perhaps the exact same players are at work. A previous injury may have created scar tissue that inhibits musculature from working properly. An abdominal weakness may not allow you to support your posture properly, and is thus the cause of your back pain. The tightness of your legs may be the reason you are having trouble bending over, or have pulled a hamstring, or have knee problems. You must determine for yourself the origins of this pain.

Pain Versus Pain

Only you can judge what pain is. As a dancer, I have an extremely high tolerance for pain. Once dancers get their bodies warm, they work through the pain and dance regardless of whether their hips are out of whack or their hamstrings are torn. That's what dancers do. They dance. Athletes work through pain in a similar fashion. Often, professional athletes will be playing in a game a week after surgery. They have pain, but they play through it. For someone who is not a professional dancer or athlete, however, pain can be a completely different issue. Everyone has a different tolerance for pain.

The first step in dealing with pain is to know the difference between the pain of an injury and the soreness in a muscle caused by working out. When you lift weights or engage in aerobic activity, you are tearing muscle tissue. The torn muscle tissue heals and becomes stronger. In this process of tearing and healing, the muscles secrete a substance called lactic acid, a crystalline substance that stays within the muscle tissue. The next time you engage in that activity, the crystalline lactic acid breaks apart and works itself out of the muscle tissue, and that is why the muscle hurts. When people have a personal trainer, the workout will oftentimes be so hard that they are in pain for several days afterward. More often than not, those people will not return to the gym because they feel like they need a sling and a pulley to lift food to their mouths. When you begin working out, it is important to get past that lactic acid or you will never get anywhere with your workout. Drinking more water can offset much of this uncomfortable feeling of soreness. You may also want to think about applying ice to the sore areas, and/or using Epsom salts as a cathartic in your bath.

This soreness is acceptable pain. Don't be afraid of it. Some people fear it because they think they have done something harmful to themselves. There is a huge difference between this kind of soreness and an injury. If, on the other hand, you are stretching or working out and you hear a muscle tear or your hamstring pop, you know you have done something harmful to your body.

The principle of weight training and aerobic exercise is that strength is gained through the body healing the muscle tissue torn and broken down during such exercise. Pilates works on a different principle altogether. You are not tearing or breaking down muscle tissue. The soreness that you may have experienced from lifting weights usually does not occur with Pilates. You will experience some soreness associated with stretching or working your musculature, but it won't be a soreness that impedes you from doing anything that you normally do. In fact, you will immediately notice that your posture and the way you carry yourself will be much improved. Your body will be holding itself differently. This can lead to a wide array of positive mental adjustments, like more confidence, readiness, and calmness, and an improved ability to deal with stress and all that life throws at you. If you are doing this routine four or five times a week, in two weeks' time you will be physically certain that you are getting in shape and getting stronger. You will feel much more flexible. In one month's time, those around you will notice that you are changing.

How Do We Injure Ourselves?

Injury and injury prevention are interrelated. To understand the main reasons for why and how we injure ourselves is to insure that we will prevent injury. The main reasons why we injure ourselves are a lack of movement consciousness, working outside the frame of the body, imbalance, lack of strength, and a lack of flexibility. When we injure ourselves, one or all of these factors are at work. One of the many benefits the Pilates method of body conditioning offers is to vastly improve these areas. The more you engage in this exercise, the less likely you are to injure yourself.

Movement Consciousness

I believe that the primary cause for injury is a lack of consciousness about the way we move. We are either not thinking about what we are doing or are not aware of how we are moving. We may move too quickly, we may jerk the body, we may twist too hard, or we may even injure ourselves while we sleep. A great example is when we see some blood on our clothes and realize we have a cut on our hand, but have no idea of when or how it happened. A pot starts slipping off the stove. You see it out of your peripheral vision and twist yourself around quickly to catch it. Later in the day, you just can't figure out why your knee is hurting, your back is out, and your shoulder is throbbing.

Movement consciousness is an awareness of where you are in time and space. This is not a New Age, see-your-guru kind of awareness. I'll give you an example. You have heard a million times, "Bend your knees when you are picking something up." I have a friend who lifts weights every day. He could lift me over his head with one arm without even thinking about it. But one day he reached over to pick up some barbells; he wasn't paying attention and, by picking them up unconsciously, threw out his back. We can save ourselves much pain and suffering by bringing a sense of awareness or mindfulness to the way we move. For some, this awareness may be elusive, but after you begin to practice this regimen, you will know exactly what I mean. It is a quality of being within yourself while at the same time being aware of your surroundings and what you're doing. In Pilates, all movement emanates from your center, inside your abdominals—the place that connects the stomach with the spine with the buttocks. From this place, you become very aware of movement and how that center supports movement in a very positive way. When you find your center, you will become much more graceful. I can close my eyes and know exactly what my arm looks like in space when I move it. Pilates develops this awareness of where you are in time and space. If you don't develop that awareness, you may continue to hurt yourself.

Working Within the Frame of the Body

In Pilates, we work inside the frame of the body. When we are standing, our legs are underneath our hips; our arms are underneath our shoulders. Our shoulders and hips "frame" the body. Our joints are supported to a large degree by our smaller muscles. When you work outside the frame of your body, your smaller muscles aren't balanced in support of your larger muscles. Once you take the weight of your joint or bone outside the frame of your body—and the body frame can no longer support it—then it's on its own. If you are not strong enough to support that movement, you risk injuring yourself.

We most often see this happen in sports. If you're playing tennis and you swing at a ball that is out of reach, the consequence is pulling your back. Basically what you have done is overextend yourself. Your body was not supporting the movement, and you got hurt. You can absolutely reduce your chances of being injured when you learn to work within the frame of your body. Pilates works exclusively within the frame of the body, which provides an environment where it is safe for the small and large muscles to work harmoniously and without putting undue weight on the joints. As you become more and more familiar with this boundary, it will be much safer to work outside this frame when you play your favorite sports.

Inflexibility

Inflexibility is also a key component to injury. The tighter we are, the less room our musculature has to move. If you are inflexible and stiff, you cannot move freely, and if you try to force it, you will increase your chances of pulling or tearing something. If you are naturally very stiff and inflexible and you exercise without stretching, you're in for trouble. If you are twenty-five years old, it might be fine to do that, but as we get older the world just doesn't work that way anymore. I have a client who said to me, "You know, I'm sixty now and all those times that I played tennis and ran and skied and jumped and played without stretching and without paying attention to my body, I'm paying for it now." His back is killing him, and he has problems with his feet and his bone strength. He tried to keep doing all the activities he had done when he was younger, but he found that his body just did not respond the way it used to. He became increasingly inflexible over the years because he did not stretch on a regular basis. As we age, inflexibility becomes our main enemy. In extreme cases, muscles can tighten up around the joint and cause arthritis. Pilates increases our flexibility each and every time we perform the routine.

Weakness

Weakness also causes injury. This is a simple concept: When we are strong, we are less likely to become injured. When I say strong, I don't mean that we can lift a locomotive over our heads like Superman. I'm very petite but am much stronger than most weight lifters coming in for the first time. The weight lifter relies almost exclusively on the larger muscles to do his kind of work. If he overuses the larger muscles without strengthening his smaller musculature, he increases his chances of injuring himself. Pilates strengthens and develops smaller muscle groups that support the larger muscles. When a weight lifter is in the gym, he may be doing a "curl" with a barbell in his hand. He is isolating the bicep muscle and trying to work that particular muscle into exhaustion. When I perform the same exercise, the movement comes from my powerhouse or center, my posture is aligned, and I am working my abdominals, my chest, my scapula, my forearm, and my wrist, as well as my bicep. With Pilates, that same weight lifter could learn to call on the smaller muscles to aid him in his work, and thus perform at much higher levels. He may be able to lift more, to do more repetitions, to surpass a plateau that he has been working at, and to see more muscular definition.

Imbalance

Imbalance in the body is another link to injury. Balance and alignment are closely related and can work as allies to help make you stronger. Balance and alignment of the body is crucial to create relief from pain and prevent injury. In most people, one side is stronger than the other. You're either right-handed or left-handed. You use your dominant hand for most strenuous activity, so that side of the body is much more developed than the other. The arm is bigger, the shoulder muscles are much more developed, and the back muscles are larger. This is an imbalance. The stronger side will eventually become sore and tender as a result of overuse. The weaker side has a tendency to atrophy. When your washing machine is out of balance, you can hear it clanking all through the house. So it is with your body. If you perform most tasks with your strong side without strengthening the weaker side, you will eventually be in a situation in which your body is out of whack. If the imbalance goes unchecked, it causes a domino effect throughout the body. Before you know it, you are completely out of alignment, and you have a variety of physical pains. If for some reason you take the limbs outside the frame of the body, the imbalance between your strong side and your weak side will almost always result in injury. This is a syndrome or pattern of imbalance that you must force yourself to break.

Almost everyone is out of balance. It is just a matter of degree. Pilates will help you balance the body, but you must be mindful of working evenly. In other words, if you are moving one leg a certain distance, you need to try to copy that same distance with the other leg. Pay close attention to your body's symmetry, also. If one leg is much stronger or more flexible than the other, you need to balance them both as you're working. In other words, work the weaker leg more than the stronger leg, and stretch the inflexible leg more than the flexible leg, until the legs are equal. In this way you discontinue the old pattern. You want to try to keep balance. After my motorcycle accident, I knew I really had to work on my entire left side. That side of my body was beginning to atrophy from inactivity. I began to strengthen and stretch that side of my body, and then and only then did I begin to feel and see the results of my hard work. The greater my achievement, the greater, almost overwhelming, sense of control I could feel. And the more control I had over my body, the greater the healing.

Movement is one of the great gifts that we as human beings were given. When we have an injury, our movement becomes limited, and as a result our quality of life is diminished. There are, however, certain things that you can do to control your own destiny. When you balance your body, you are doing something extraordinarily healthy for yourself. When you are in balance, you are in harmony with yourself and the world around you. A significant mental facet of movement develops. The mental aspect of healing, and of movement in general, improves the quality of your life in ways you may not even be aware of. Your body and your entire system is able to work more efficiently and at a higher level. When operating on this higher level, you can live your life passionately and euphorically. You become part of a very positive force. You are working with the powers that be. You are working with joy.

Neck Injuries

Let's first talk about what I mean by a bad neck. I am not talking about injuries that have anything to do with bones. If you have been in a car accident and are wearing a neck brace, you need a more professional, hands-on, opinion. Similarly, if you have chronic neck problems, it is best to consult with a doctor or physical therapist, or to see a chiropractor, because it may mean that your neck is out of alignment. If Pilates is not enough to bring it back into alignment, you need to see a professional, if only to get an evaluation. The bottom line is that you do not want to engage in any activity that will make the problem worse. What I refer to as a "bad neck" involves a much less severe variation of pain, and can be attributed to a number of things. You may have slept "funny," you may have turned too quickly, you may have been cradling the phone with your shoulder or lifting heavy objects above your head. It can even be caused by tension or stress. Because there are so many probable causes for this pain, I simply cannot make a judgment on why you are experiencing it. What we are talking about is the inability to move in a full range of motion.

In Chapter 5, on the mat work routine, you may have noted that there were several exercises you should not do if you have a BAD NECK: The Roll-Over, Criss-Cross, Open Leg Rocker, Scissors, Bicycle, Jackknife, The Boomerang, and The Seal. These exercises require you to roll back onto your neck or to twist your neck in a manner that may be uncomfortable.

If what you have is a stiff neck, you may perform the rest of the routine with some minor adjustments. In Rolling Like a Ball, DO NOT roll back onto your neck. When you are doing the Single Leg Stretch, the Double Leg Stretch, the Single Straight Leg, and the Double Straight Leg, rest your head on a pillow. I recommend that you do not do these exercises with a flat neck, as it will be too unstable or uncomfortable for you. The Side Kick Series may be adjusted in the following way: Instead of propping your head

---

This chapter outlines some exercises that you can do for a bad neck.

up on top of your hand, bend the elbow and lay the arm out against the mat, then lay your head on top of the folded arm. Any exercise that specifies that you lift your head off the mat may be traumatic. In these cases, try not to hold the head up using your neck muscles.

The following are some fantastic exercises that you can perform that will loosen and stretch the muscles in your neck. I recommend that you perform these exercises if you feel any discomfort in your neck or before beginning the mat routine.

Dr. Robert Forrester's Neck Stretch

Ready

Sit straight up with
your legs crossed in front of you.

Action

Place the palm of your right hand on the mat,
with your fingers pointed toward you.
Now sit on your hand.
Extend your left arm straight up to the ceiling
directly above your shoulder.
Curve your arm over your head,
and *gently* pull your head toward your left
shoulder.
Feel the stretch along the right side of
your neck.
Come back to center, and repeat on the
other side.

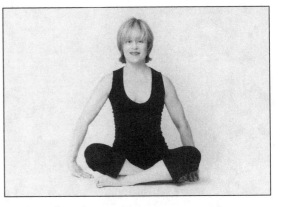

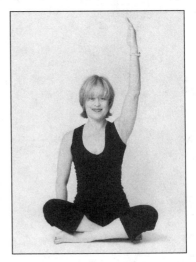

This exercise was not designed by Joseph Pilates.

Sit on your left hand.
Turn your head slightly, and
relax your head toward your right shoulder,
pointing your nose toward the armpit.
Bring the right hand over the top of your
head, and let it rest on the back of your head.
Let the weight of your right arm stretch your
neck, as your right elbow releases down
toward the mat.
Breathe into the stretch.
Pull into the powerhouse and deepen the
stretch.
With your head at this 45-degree angle,
release your arm and
bring your head slowly back to center.

Repeat on the other side.
Do 3 sets.

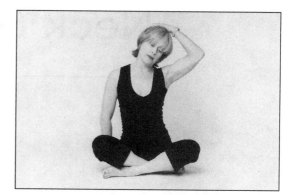

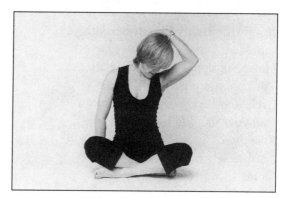

Neck Stretch

Ready

Lie on your stomach.

Action

Bring your hands directly beneath your
shoulders.
Glue your upper thighs to the mat.
Push up, straighten your arms.
Arch your back as much as you can.
Pull your shoulders down.
Stay there.
Look slowly to your right.
Come back to center.
Look slowly to your left.
Come back to center.
Repeat.

Tilt your head toward your right shoulder.
Come back to center.
Tilt your head toward your left shoulder.
Come back to center.
Relax your chin toward your chest.
Come back to center.
Repeat twice.

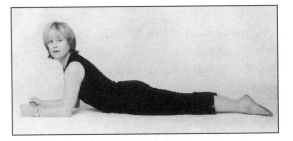

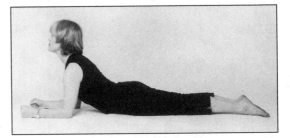

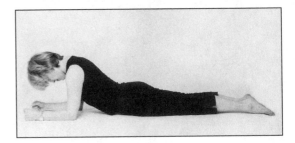

Chest Expansion

Ready

Kneel on the mat with your legs together.
Your chest should feel lifted.
Your arms extend straight out in a
sleepwalking position.
Pull in from the powerhouse to
lengthen through your spine.

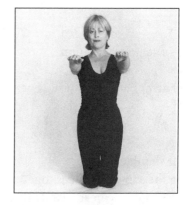

Action

Push your arms straight back,
like you are pushing wet cement,
past your buttocks.
Push your arms back as far as they will go,
so you are open across your chest,
and hold that position.
Keep your shoulders down.
Look to the right.
Come back to center.
Look to the left.
Come back to center.
Release your arms down to your sides.

Repeat 5–10 times.

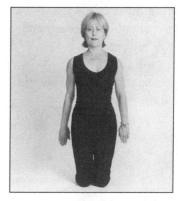

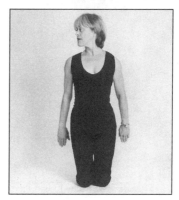

Shoulder Circles

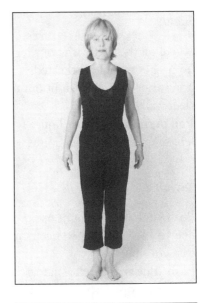

Ready

Come to a standing position.
Lengthen the spine.
Let your arms hang comfortably at your side.

Action

Pull your shoulders back,
tweezing the shoulder blades together in back.
Lift your shoulders up and circle them forward
as you bring them up toward your ears.
Circle your shoulders forward and
bring them back around.
If you had paintbrushes
sticking straight out of your shoulders,
you could paint circles.

Repeat 5 times.

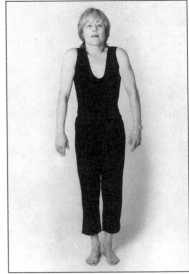

This exercise was not designed by Joseph Pilates.

Come back to center.
Now reverse the circle.
Push your shoulders forward.
Circle up,
pulling your shoulders up toward your ears.
Circle back,
tweezing the shoulder blades together.

Repeat 5 times.

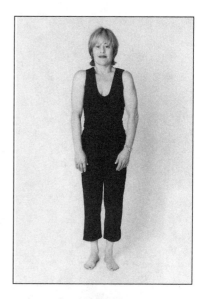

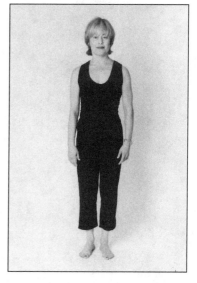

Lower Back Pain and Weakness

This discussion will be limited specifically to the lower back. You should seek professional advice if you are experiencing constant pain.

The lower back is an area that you can improve with work. The lower back pain I am talking about has links to numerous causes: stress, muscle tightness, improper posture, and misalignment. We can strain or injure the lower back by lifting heavy objects, or lifting those objects improperly. If we sit for extended periods of time, or do not stretch regularly, we can sometimes feel compressed in this area; in these cases, simple stretching can be very helpful.

There are several exercises in the mat work routine in Chapter 5 that I DO NOT recommend if you have a bad lower back, specifically the Roll-Over, the Corkscrew, and the Criss-Cross should be avoided. These exercises generally require you to twist the body. There are other exercises you should gradually work up toward, or make the movements very small at first and then gradually, over time, let them become more dynamic. For the most part, you will have to be the judge. If any of these exercises make you nervous, DO NOT DO THEM.

Pilates can help the lower back in three areas and help to alleviate any discomfort associated with them. The three areas (which are interrelated and affect each other a great deal) that Pilates concentrates on are ensuring proper alignment and proper posture, strengthening the abdominal muscles, and increasing the flexibility of the hamstrings. Most doctors recommend that you strengthen abdominal muscles to alleviate lower back pain. Not only is strength in this region of the body a key factor in our ability to move, but it is also the key to proper alignment of the spine. Proper placement of the spine, especially within the lower back, is dependent upon the strength of the abdominal muscles, and much of the Pilates method is focused on strengthening the abdominal musculature. Flexibility is often a key issue. When you first begin using the Pilates method of body conditioning, you may notice that you are especially tight in the legs, especially in the area of the hamstrings, which may be related to your lower back pain.

You may do most of the exercises in the mat work, but with slight adjustments, most of which concern placement of the legs. For the sake of your lower back, pay close attention to the directions concerning leg placement. When you are on your back, adjust the directions so that the small of your back is in constant contact with the mat. If the directions call for the legs to be extended straight out from the hips, you may have to bring your knees into your chest, or bend your knees and put your feet flat on the mat. Do only what you can do without the small of your back losing contact with the mat. Other exercises are performed lying on the stomach. When you are lying on your stomach, place a pillow underneath your pelvis for support.

The remainder of this chapter takes you through several exercises. We begin with some basic breathing exercises that will work on your alignment; they focus on the ability of the powerhouse, or abdominal musculature, to strengthen the lower back. We then move on to some modifications to the beginning mat work. Finally, there are specific exercises for bad backs. If you suffer from a bad back, do these exercises until you become fairly proficient at them, then slowly work your way into the mat work using the demonstrated modifications. Over time, move closer to the directions as stated, and then proceed to the intermediate and advanced stages. When you make the jump from beginning to intermediate, you should have achieved sufficient muscle strength to alleviate your lower back pain.

Lower Back Stretch

This is a simple stretch for the back. You should perform it before you begin any activity.

Ready

Lie on your back.
Slowly bring your feet in toward your buttocks.
Feel you whole spine against the mat.
Breathe and relax.

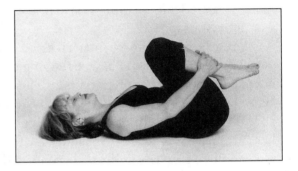

Action

Gently bring your knees up
and hug them into your chest.
Release some tension in your arms and
cross your ankles.
Hug your knees in again.
Your back is long against the mat.
Repeat 10 times.
Release your hands and unhook your ankles.
Leave your legs right where they are.
Feel that your lower back is pressed into
the mat.
Just stay there and feel your lower back
lengthen.
Breathe.
Pull your powerhouse in toward your lower
back, and then squeeze your buttocks
together to lengthen even further,
and to increase the muscular support for
your lower back.

For right now, you want your lower back against the mat. If you are performing any of these exercises and feel your back arching or coming off the mat, do whatever you have to do to get back the feeling of being against the mat.

Modified Hundred

With this exercise, we warm up the body with breath and with movement.
When you are finished, you should feel warmth around the heart area.

Prep

Lie on your back.
Feel your whole spine meet the floor.
Your spine is long and open.
Your arms are long against your body.
Palms are face down, flat on the mat.
Knees are pointed to the ceiling.
Feet are flat on the mat.

Ready

Using the powerhouse, bring your chin into
your chest.
DO NOT lift the upper body higher than
the base of the shoulder blades.

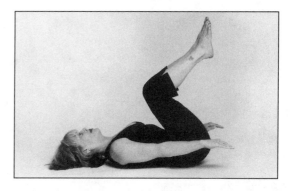

Action

Pull the powerhouse
tightly into your lower back.
Inhale slowly through the nose for 5 counts
while pumping your arms up and down.
Your arms are rigid,
like a hammer pounding a nail.
Exhale slowly through the nose for 5 counts,
continuing to pump the arms up and down.
Pull that powerhouse in.

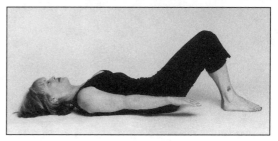

Keep your arms straight.
Keep only your arms and shoulders involved
in the movement.

Repeat the cycle until
you have counted up to 100.
Relax completely.

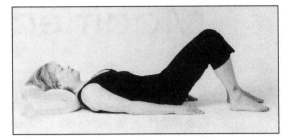

Modified Roll-Up

This exercise will really put you in touch with your powerhouse. The powerhouse connects everything—try to feel that connection as you do this exercise.

Ready

While sitting up tall,
place your feet flat on the mat
with your knees pointing toward the ceiling.
Place the palms of your hands underneath
your thighs and point your elbows away from
your body.

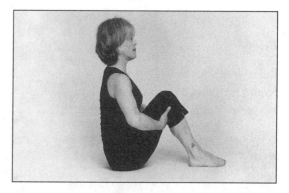

Action

Pull your navel into your spine.
Let that contraction curve your lower back
into the shape of a "C."
Roll back into the contraction
until your arms are straight.
Pull your powerhouse in even further.
Pull with your arms and your powerhouse,
NOT WITH YOUR BACK.

Repeat 6–8 times.

As you feel your abdominal muscles
becoming stronger, do the same movement
without your arms, using only the
powerhouse.

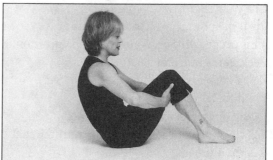

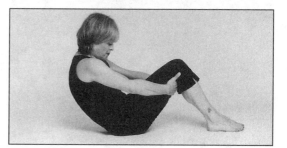

Dr. Grode's Stomach Exercise

This is a wonderful exercise to strengthen the abdominal muscles, and to lengthen the spine.

Ready

Relax your legs down.
Knees are bent, feet flat on the mat.
Kneecaps are pointed toward the ceiling.

Action

Cross your arms across your chest.
Lift your chin toward your chest.
Push the powerhouse into your spine.
This isn't a "crunch"—just hold the position.
Feel your spine elongate.
Relax your neck.
Hold for 20 counts.
Push your navel toward your spine.
Slowly relax your head back down to the mat.
Repeat 4 times.

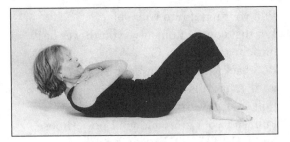

This exercise was not designed by Joseph Pilates.

Oppositional Stretch

Ready

Lie flat on your back.
Your left arm is extended straight out,
resting flat on the mat
so that it is perpendicular to your torso and
with your fingers pointing away from you.

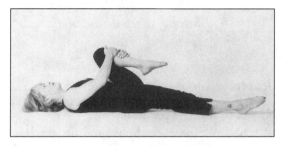

Action

Hug your left knee into your chest
with your right hand.
Draw that leg toward your right side.
Rest your left foot on top of your right thigh.
Turn your head to look at your left hand.
If this feels comfortable,
bring your knee down toward the mat.

Repeat on your other side.

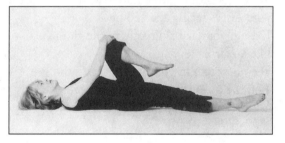

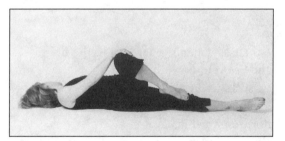

This exercise was not designed by Joseph Pilates.

The Saw

This exercise will stretch the hamstrings, the waist, and the lower back very effectively. Keep the buttocks firmly planted on the mat to maximize this stretch.

Ready

Come to a sitting position.
Lift up from the powerhouse and sit up tall.
Your legs should be shoulder-width apart with your knees facing the ceiling.
Extend your arms directly to the side,
like an airplane,
keeping them in your peripheral sight.
Pull the powerhouse into your lower back.
Your shoulders are pressing down toward the lats.

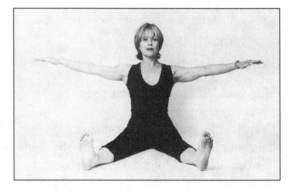

Action

Exhale as you glue your butt to the floor,
and use your powerhouse to
twist slowly to the right.
Twist gently from your waist,
not from the hips.
Reach your left pinky toward the right little toe.
(Your right arm will drop when it gets behind you.)
Stretch your body forward.
Your head reaches over your right knee.
Relax your neck,
and keep the opposite hip down.
Exhale slowly
as you perform 3 saw-like pulses.

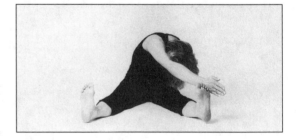

Saw that little toe off.
Stretch from your waist.
Complete the exhalation.
—From the powerhouse—
Roll up and return to center.
Repeat on the left side.
Do 4 sets.

Little Piece of Heaven

If your knees hurt when you are rounded over, simply place a pillow between your buttocks and your heels.

Ready

You are still lying on your stomach.

Action

Use your hands and arms to
push yourself back onto your heels
until you are kneeling with your back
rounded over.
Focus on the mat.
Extend your arms long in front of you.
Push your hips to your heels
for a deep lower back stretch.
Breathe slowly and deeply.
Rest the back.

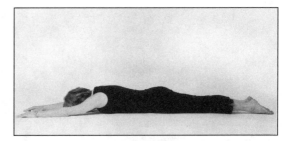

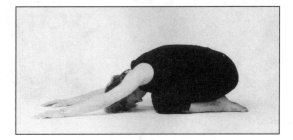

Rolling Down the Wall

This is a wonderful exercise to finish the session. This exercise will really stretch out the lower back.

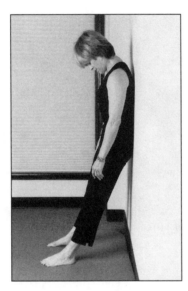

Ready

Come to a standing position
with your back against the wall.
Your feet are hip-width apart,
about 1 foot away from the wall.
Feel your entire spine against the wall,
keeping your shoulders open.

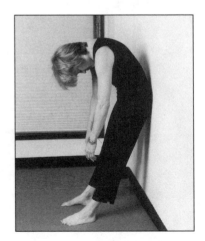

Action

Slowly let your head drop forward.
When your chin nears your chest,
feel the weight of your head
begin to lead you down.
Pull your ribs in and continue to stretch your
neck and upper back.
Pull the powerhouse in toward your spine.
Relax your entire upper body; let the weight of
your head, neck, and upper body pull you over.
You may even have to bend your knees slightly.
Scoop your pelvis underneath you.
Slide your pelvis up the wall
as you straighten your legs.
Press your lower back against the wall.
Pull the powerhouse in as you
roll up, vertebra by vertebra,
until you are upright.

Repeat 3 times.

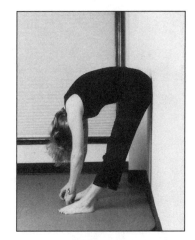

Asthma

CHAPTER 9

There are only two rules when you have asthma:

1. Always, and I do mean *always*, carry your inhaler with you at all times.
2. If you have an attack doing Pilates, or any other activity, *stop*.

Asthma remains somewhat of a mystery. There is so much that we do not know about this condition. Although science has told us much, asthma continues to baffle health professionals and researchers. Although the inventor of this method of body conditioning, Joseph Pilates, was himself an asthmatic, and designed these exercises to alleviate his own condition, there have been no scientific studies on how the Pilates exercise affects asthmatics and what benefits it can offer asthma sufferers. I can only relay my own personal experience. I can state unequivocally that it has helped me immensely. I can honestly say that I cannot remember the last time I had a full-blown "attack." Yes, I can be heard to wheeze on occasion, but even that has improved over the years. This does not mean that I have thrown away my inhaler—I still carry it with me everywhere I go. I am not without asthma, but I have found that through this series of exercises I can control it, and it does not control me.

It has been my experience that asthma is induced mainly by stress or exercise. In my case, I believe it is more often stress-related, and exercise has really helped me relieve some of that stress. If your asthma tends to be stress-related, the exercises in this section should work well for you. If, on the other hand, your asthma is exercise-induced, you must consult your doctor to get advice on breathing techniques, or have him or her look over the following exercises.

Breathing is, of course, fundamental to living, and is thus also fundamental in movement. Since in this book we are talking specifically about moving, the way in which you breathe when you perform this routine will not only advance your progress in this method of conditioning, but it could help your breathing in general. If we somehow forget to breathe when we are moving, or we take on a strenuous task and hold our breath while doing it, the body has a tendency to tense up. For instance, I have found that if I do not warm up properly before I exercise, I can stress my body and bring on my asthma. This is the physiological reaction when the muscles are not receiving enough oxygen. When oxygen can reach the muscles, the body gains the ability to relax—the muscles elongate and they are able to stretch. Combining focused movement with breathing is the key to elongating the musculature. The more we can oxygenate and elongate the musculature, the less stress we have within the body. The less stress we have within the body, the more we can alleviate our asthma.

You can clearly see the advantages of taking in a full breath, but exhalation is just as important. When we exhale, we expel nonbeneficial gasses and other toxins stored within the body. In a crude way, exhaling is almost like flushing a toilet. It is one of the primary ways the human body disposes of what is unhealthy. This full exhalation is what we referred to in Chapter 3 as "wringing out the lungs." The more fully we can exhale, the more air we can take in. To use an analogy, if the lungs were a waterlogged sponge, that sponge would not be able to absorb any more water. If we wring the sponge out until it is almost dry, not only do we dispose of the dirty water, but the sponge would be able to absorb a great quantity of new water.

When we move, our breath can take on a life of its own. I have observed in singers and musicians that where and when they breathe fuels the music. As a dancer, I have experienced the breath truly linking one movement to the next. The breath acts as a gel for the performer. In the arts, they define this as "organic"—meaning that the work transcends mere notes of music or carefully choreographed movements, and enters into the spirit of the performer. If breath can be the gel for performers, allowing their whole being to be fully involved with the work on many different levels, even relaying the passion of the spirit, the same is certainly true of the breath as it relates to Pilates. Bodily coordination is certainly emphasized with this technique, but it is truly the breath that allows us to achieve our intended goals in movement. Having asthma makes breathing in this way all the more challenging.

For the asthma sufferer, breathing will be a little different than it is described for the mat work exercises. In the following pages, you will find some exercises that I have found to be quite remarkable. I would recommend that you concentrate not so much on the inhalation, but on the exhalation. For these exercises, it is vital that you expel as much air as you can. If you inhale for two counts, I want you to exhale for six counts. Let's try it with some basic breathing exercises. These exercises may be practiced before you begin the routine, or at any other time during the day. I use them to offset wheezing, and I have found that they help me prepare my body for movement. These exercises allow you to take in more breath, reduce muscular tension, and, hopefully, will help you offset your asthmatic condition.

Wringing Out
the Lungs

Begin by doing this simple breathing exercise to emphasize the technique we were just discussing.

Ready

Place a pillow under your head.
Lie flat on your back.
Knees are bent, feet are flat on the mat.
Kneecaps are pointed toward the ceiling.

Action

Inhale for 2 full counts.
Exhale forcefully for 6 counts.
Inhale for 2 full counts,
and exhale for 6 as you
add a little sound—SHHHHHHHHHHH.
Inhale for 2 counts as you
relax the legs flat against the mat.
Exhale for 6 counts—SHHHHHHHHHHH.

Repeat 10 times.

Modified Hundred

This is a modified version of the exercise of the same name found in the mat routine. The movements are exactly the same, only the breathing cadence is changed. With this exercise, we warm up the body with breath and with movement. When you finish, you should feel warmth around the heart area.

Prep

Lie on your back.
Feel your whole spine meet the floor.
The spine is long and open.
Arms are long against your body.
Palms are face down and flat on the mat.
Knees are pointed to the ceiling.
Feet are flat on the mat.

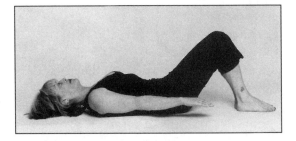

Ready

Using the powerhouse, bring your chin into your chest.
DO NOT lift the upper body higher than the base of the shoulder blades.

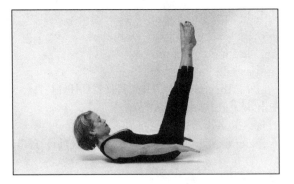

Action

Pull the powerhouse tightly into your
lower back.
Inhale slowly through your nose for 3 counts
while pumping your arms up and down.
Your arms are rigid.
Think of them as hammers pounding on a nail.
Exhale slowly through your nose for 7 counts,
continuing to pump your arms up and down.
Get all that air out.
Pull that powerhouse in.
Keep your arms straight.
Keep only your arms and shoulders involved
in the movement.
Repeat the cycle until
you have counted up to 100.
Relax completely.

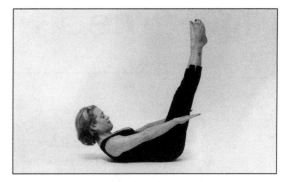

Modified Footwork #1

This is the first of three breathing exercises involving footwork. This exercise can also be performed in a Pilates studio utilizing an apparatus called the Reformer. On this apparatus, your feet would be pushing against a bar that is connected to a number of springs that create a resistance for the movement. When performing this exercise on the mat, it is essential that you mimic this resistance to the movement.

Ready

Place the pillow back under your head.
Lie flat on your back.
Feel the small of your back against the mat,
with your arms rest comfortably at your side,
palms are against the mat.
Hug your knees into your chest
and release your hands,
keeping your legs where they are.
Open your knees until
they are even with your shoulders.
Your heels are together, your toes are apart.

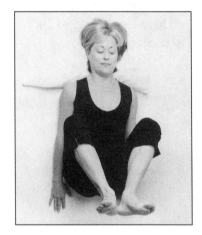

Action

Push your legs toward the point where
the ceiling and the wall meet.
Push your legs
as if you were moving through wet cement.
Your legs are now at a 45-degree angle.
If you have a bad back,
lift your legs straight up toward the ceiling.

Maintain the same foot position
as you release your knees back
toward your shoulders,
again moving through imaginary cement,
creating resistance in the movement.
Now let's layer the breathing into this.
Inhale as you
push the legs out and pull them back in.
(This completes 1 set.)
Exhale and complete 3 or 4 sets
(depending on your lung capacity).
Don't throw your legs.
You want the movement to have dynamic,
but you do need resistance as well.

Repeat 10 times.

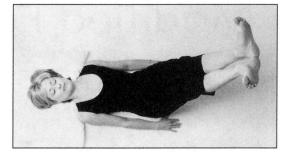

Modified Footwork #2

Ready

End the last series as your
knees come back toward your shoulders.
Bring your knees and ankles together.
Curl your toes down toward the mat.

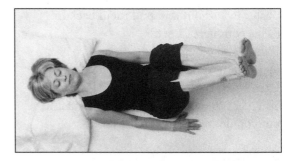

Action

Inhale for 2 counts as you
push your legs out at a 45-degree angle
and bring them back into the body,
to complete 1 set.
Again imagine you are moving the legs
through wet cement.
Exhale through 3 or 4 sets.
Repeat 5 times.

Modified Footwork #3

Ready

Flex your toes back toward your body.
Glue your knees and ankles together.
Lift your legs so that your heels are even with
your knees.

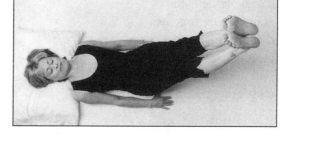

Action

Inhale as you
push your heels, as if moving through wet
cement, toward the point where the ceiling
and the wall meet.
Bring your knees back into your chest.
Exhale as you complete 3 or 4 additional sets.
Repeat 5 times.

Chest Expansion

Ready

Kneel on the mat.
Your legs are together.
Bring your arms up into a sleepwalking
position.
Pull in from the powerhouse to
lengthen through your spine.

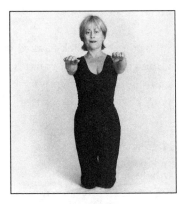

Action

Inhale.
Push your arms straight back,
like you are pushing wet cement
past your buttocks.
Push your arms back as far as they will go
so that you are open across the chest.
Hold that position.
Keep your shoulders down.
Hold your breath as you look to the right.
Come back to center.
Look to the left.
Come back to center.
Exhale as you release your arms through the
cement and back to center.
Repeat 10 times.

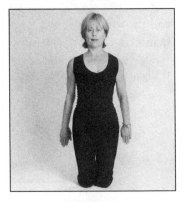

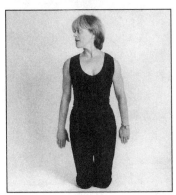

Modified Neck Roll

The object of this exercise is to open the chest and the airways.

Prep

Release your body down to the mat.
Gently roll over onto your stomach.

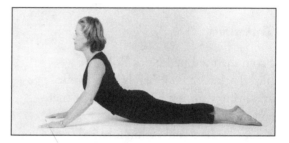

Action

Exhale as you
bring your hands directly beneath your
shoulders.
Glue your upper thighs to the mat.
Push up.
Arch your back as much as you can.
Pull your shoulders down.
Stay there.

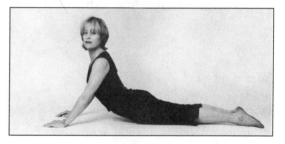

If you are flexible, keep your hips on the mat.
Inhale deeply as you
lift your head slowly toward the point
where the ceiling and wall meet.
Exhale as you
bring your head back to center.
Repeat 2 times.

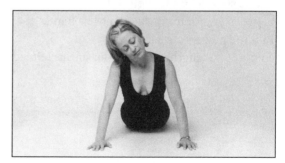

The Mermaid

This exercise is designed to open the lungs across the chest, across the back, and along the sides.

Transition

From the modified Neck Roll,
push back with your hands, bend your knees,
and bring your left hip down to the mat,
so you are sitting on that hip.
Knees are bent and facing forward (right knee
on top of the left, right foot on top of the left).

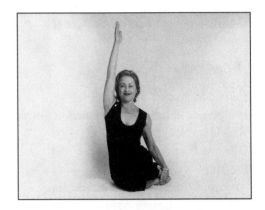

Ready

Your right hand
holds your right ankle for balance.
Stretch your left arm
straight up above your shoulder.
There should be a straight line
between your left hip and your left hand.
Pull the powerhouse in and
continue to lengthen along your entire left side.

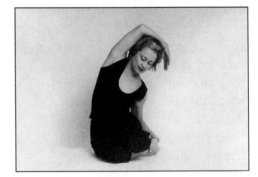

Action

Let your left arm fall over your head
and reach your body toward the right side.
Feel the stretch throughout the ribs on your
left side.
Extend your left arm straight up again.
Pull the shoulders down. Your neck is long.
Reach your left hand down to the mat,
fingers pointing away from you.
Stretch the right arm up and over your head,
fingers toward the ceiling.
Pull the powerhouse into your spine.
Lengthen.
Lean to your left and let your elbow bend.
Stretch straight out to the left side,
as far as you can without coming off the mat.
Push up from your forearm,
and come back to center.
Come up onto your knees
and sit on your right hip.
Repeat on other side.
Repeat this exercise 2 more times.

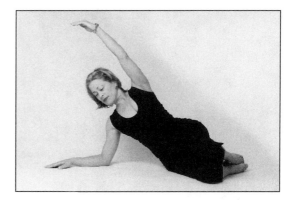

Beyond the Mat

Up to this point, you have worked on becoming extremely strong—especially within the powerhouse—and improving your control and coordination of movement. You could continue work with the mat routine, be perfectly satisfied that you are being challenged, and never become bored with the routine. However, you may feel like you would like to advance to a higher level in this method of body conditioning.

This chapter offers some options for such advancement. Topics we will discuss include exercise devices developed by Joseph Pilates; finding a studio that has the proper apparatus; questions that you should ask your trainer before you begin working out; and information on how Pilates instructors become certified. I will introduce you to the man who is responsible for the certification process, and let him give you some insight into how health care professionals are making Pilates part of the physical therapy healing regimen.

When you perform the mat work, you are working with the resistance and the strength of your own body. It's just you and your body. On the other hand, when you do this work on equipment specifically designed for the movement, the equipment accents all the resistance-oriented exercises that you're doing, allowing you to have even more resistance. Instead of "moving through wet cement," as I have often suggested, springs or pulleys provide that resistance. Because this resistance is non-weight-bearing, you are not pumping or gasping for air, and, as in the mat routine, this limits the possibility of injury. The equipment may allow you to take the mat work a step further, and it may even help you develop musculature faster.

On your first visit to a Pilates Studio®, you may be a little intimidated by the array of devices confronting you. Have no fear, the exercises that you will be doing on the apparatus will be similar to exercises you have been doing on the mat. The equipment's basic functions are to create greater resistance, and enable you to have a deeper stretch. It may be helpful to introduce you to the apparatus so that will be familiar with their names and functions if you do decide that you would like to try them.

The first device that you would encounter at a Pilates studio would be The Reformer. This is the main piece of equipment in a studio, the workhorse. This apparatus was probably fashioned from a bed. It is rectangular in shape, stands about 12 inches off the floor, and is about 7 feet long. On top of the frame is a 4-foot-long padded board that you lie on. This board is on a carriage that can slide the entire length of the frame. The frame is capable of transforming itself with cables, springs, and pulleys into many shapes, and it can accommodate many body positions. With minor adjustments, most of the mat routine can be done on this machine.

Another device is The Cadillac. This has about the same proportions as The Reformer, except that the bed is 4 feet off the ground, and it does not have a movable carriage. Designed like a canopy bed, it is close to 9 feet tall. An array of straps, springs, and pulleys can be attached and used to provide buoyancy and resistance for the legs. I believe that Pilates was inspired to build this by clients who were hospitalized and in traction. This device is my personal favorite. I have found it very helpful to attain deep stretching and in toning musculature.

Joseph Pilates was a circus performer, and many of his early devotees were also from the circus. The materials for the equipment had to be readily available, easy to transport, and also had to be functional when not in use as training equipment. A perfect example is another important piece of equipment, The Wunda Chair. When not in use as a training device, The Wunda Chair could be used at your kitchen table. When it is turned upside-down and the seat is folded back, however, it can be fitted with a vast array of springs, which instantly transforms it into one of the most advanced pieces of Pilates equipment. Some of the exercises that you have been practicing can be modified to work with The Wunda Chair.

Pilates studios usually also include two barrel-shaped devices used primarily for deep stretching. The padded Spine Corrector Barrel sits about 2 feet off the ground. This device is fantastic for people with scoliosis and osteoporosis because of the stretches you can do on it. It is also a highly effective way to find the strength in your powerhouse and your stomach that would allow optimal support. The Spine Corrector Barrel provides the least diversity, in terms of the number of exercises that it is designed for, but, when you are working with the conditions just mentioned, this piece of equipment is irreplaceable. The other barrel, The High Barrel, is actually a ladder, with the padded barrel on top. It resembles the "horse" used in gymnastics events. This apparatus is used for a very advanced series of exercises and for deep stretching.

Each one of these devices has many exercises specifically designed for it. Since you are now familiar with the principles of this method of body conditioning, the philosophy will not be foreign to your way of thinking and working. What will be somewhat different will be working with equipment. The mat work you are learning to master will help you to trust yourself and trust your body. This mastery is really a result of the mind and the body becoming one. When you work on the apparatus you have to learn to become one with the device, and to let the straps, springs, and pulleys be extensions of your own limbs. This takes some getting used to, and you should really have a professional trainer there to guide you.

How to Find a Pilates Studio

I am amazed by just how many Pilates studios are out there now. What was once a fairly obscure method of body conditioning is now becoming a real force within the fitness community. In most large communities, there should be someplace or someone available to train you. The best way to find a trainer or studio in your area is to call 1-800-4PILATE. This number connects you to The Pilates Studio of New York, which is owned and operated by Sean Gallagher and my mentor, Romana Kryznowska. These people certify Pilates trainers around the world, and they can refer you to a certified trainer in your area. If there is not a studio in your area, they can even give you names of people who have gone through the certification program who may have the equipment in their homes.

If you find a teacher who is not certified through the Pilates Studio of New York, it's important that you ask him or her some questions. Because people are not certified doesn't necessarily mean that they are poor teachers, but you want to know a few things about their qualifications to teach you. Where did they study? What is their background? Do they have a background in physical fitness? Do they have a background as a dancer? These things are really, really important. The more expertise in physical training a person has in his or her background, the more adept he or she usually is at passing on physical information. You'll want to make sure that the person didn't learn what they know from a book or a video and has at least studied with a certified teacher. Find out all their credentials. It doesn't hurt to ask. It is *your* body.

On the other hand, being certified doesn't necessarily mean that somebody's an effective teacher. It takes a really special person to be a good teacher. You may find a trainer who is a fabulous teacher, but he or she may not have all the correct information that you need. Conversely, you may find a trainer with all the information that you need, but he or she may not be an effective teacher.

You may find a Pilates instructor who is also a physical therapist. Pilates and physical therapy work very well together, since they are both primarily concerned with aligning the body and strengthening weak areas. Physical therapy can help you begin to move after an accident or surgery, and it is a natural progression to engage in "normal" activities or healing regimens that require you to become more active. Once your condition has improved to this point, traditional physical therapists will have you working with weights. Others, who may be more progressive, would have you performing Pilates exercises. Pilates makes much more sense to me because it is not weight-bearing, and it decreases your chances of aggravating or re-injuring the body part in question.

Pilates and Physical Therapy

It is only appropriate that this book end with the topic of physical therapy and Pilates. The last word on this subject comes from an interview meeting I had with Sean Gallagher. As I mentioned in the Introduction of the book, Sean is a very talented and adept physical therapist and is also the founder of the Pilates Studio of

New York. Sean is responsible for maintaining the integrity of Joseph Pilates's work and for training and certifying Pilates instructors. His unique orientation to this work made him the ideal person to talk to about this particular subject.

Sean believes that Joseph Pilates may have arguably been the first actual physical therapist. "When Joe started training, there was no such thing as physical therapy," Sean began. He told me that the profession actually began after World War I, when servicemen began returning home as amputees. "The health care workers who worked with these men were originally called reconstructive aides, and the physical therapy program as we now know it emanated from their work. By that time, Joe had been working with injuries for years. The present field of physical therapy is just beginning to realize what Joe Pilates had been practicing seventy years ago. They are beginning to do lumbar stabilization, incorporate sequential movements, concentrate on increasing the patient's strength from the center, focus on balance, and deal with balance mechanisms. Joe did all that seventy years ago."

Sean first became aware of the Pilates Method as he was finishing a dual degree in dance and in physical therapy. "When I was first exposed to this work, I had a lot of experience in physical therapy, rehabilitation, and the role that weight training has in that process. I was surprised to discover and realize that this was a system that was far superior to anything that I had been learning in school regarding physical therapy. When I returned to my teachers with this wonderful discovery, I was astounded that they had never heard of it. I began to study how applicable it was for the general population, and quickly realized that the Pilates method of body conditioning was, by far, the better system of rehabilitation for the normal person, and the normal body. I came to the conclusion that Pilates had the potential to be one of the best adjuncts for physical therapy when it comes to exercise."

When asked what makes the Pilates Method of Body Conditioning so unique and beneficial for rehabilitation, Sean replied, "Most physical therapy involves exercise. The Pilates method is extremely beneficial for both a conditioning program and for adjunct physical therapy, because you can isolate a body part if you need to. You can work on a shoulder, an elbow, or a knee. Traditional orthopedics works only on the injured area, and this work [Pilates] tends to strengthen the whole. In other words, if you had hurt your elbow, traditional orthopedics would work only on the elbow. The Pilates method works from the inside out and the elbow is connected to the shoulder, the shoulder is connected to the rib cage, the rib cage is connected to the pelvis, and movement emanates from that center. That is the way the body is designed to work. The Pilates method is much more organic than traditional exercise in that it strengthens your normal developmental sequencing process, meaning that it hooks into the way we are wired to move."

Gallagher closes on this note: "I put it in these terms: Aerobics is only twenty years old, and they are still trying to get it right. Perhaps in another fifty years, someone will have invented a good aerobics program that isn't painful or stressful on the body. In my mind, Joseph Pilates was the inventor of modern exercise. He trained all of the dancers and ballet dancers of the period, and in turn, those people taught others to move. That is the real lineage of aerobics as a form of exercise. With the mat work described in this book, and on all the [Pilates] machines, the Pilates method offers over five hundred separate exercises. In the end, this method offers such a wide variety that you can never become bored by the routine of exercise. Joe was a true genius. The methods he created eighty years ago are just now beginning to be appreciated as the groundbreaking and revolutionary work that it is. The Pilates method is so much more than an exercise regimen, it is a way of thinking and a way of life."